'Trust me, I'm a Doctor'

The Life of Victor Richard Ratten

To Margie

'Trust me, I'm a Doctor'
The Life of Victor Richard Ratten

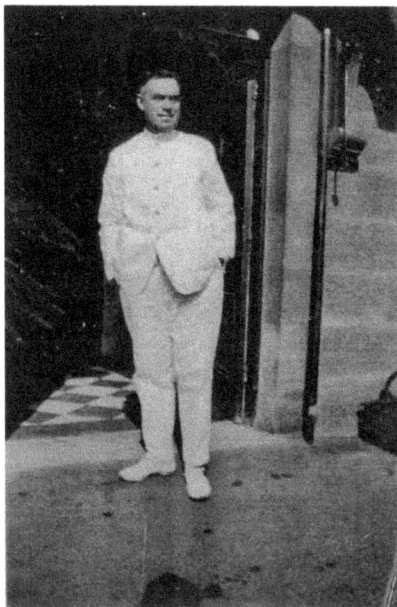

Michael Hodgson AM

Foreword

I AM delighted to offer a foreword to this book by Dr Michael Hodgson, a good friend and professional colleague. I write, like the author himself, as a senior medical clinician and historian, and as one who also has held national appointments in medical administration.

The author brings to bear extensive professional experience of medical leadership roles in the Australian Medical Association, the Australian and New Zealand College of Anaesthetists and the Australian Council on Health Care Standards, in addition to other senior State and Federal appointments, notably as President of the Medical Council of Tasmania.

In the context of this biography of Dr Victor Ratten, the author has the authority, of his extensive personal experience both in medical administration and in clinical medicine, to analyse and comment on the intriguing life of this complex medical man.

The story, hitherto untold, of the life of Dr Victor Ratten is one of the most intriguing in the history of medicine in Australia. It tells the story of a young Melbourne man who worked as an unqualified dentist in various parts of Australia; who spent eight months in the United States; and who obtained a medical 'degree' from one of the unrecognised medical colleges in Chicago which had been closed for two years. Armed with a diploma from the Harvey Medical College, in 1908 Victor Ratten set up in medical practice in Sheffield, a rural town on the north-west coast of Tasmania. After a period of militia service, Captain Ratten served for several months in the Australian Army Medical Corps before moving to Hobart where in 1916 he bought a retiring doctor's practice.

In the first decade of the twentieth century, when Victor Ratten attempted to enter the world of medicine, doctors in that post-Federation era jealously guarded their standards of training and their professional status in society. One reads of the early medical practitioners of Tasmania who at the time of the action of this biography, 'were organising themselves and flexing their muscles'.

Dr Ratten was appointed as the Surgeon Superintendent of the Hobart General Hospital in May 1917, and served in that role for the ensuing 19 years until 1936. This was a period of turbulent service, terminated by the Superintendent taking voluntary retirement under less than favourable circumstances.

Dr Ratten's turbulent professional and social life included major conflicts with the British Medical Association, the Tasmanian Medical Council and the practising clinicians of Hobart. By contrast, he was supported by members of the judiciary. He was popular both with the public and his patients and also with the nursing staff of the Hobart General Hospital. He was embroiled in numerous medico-legal proceedings, and his initial registration to practise was saved by the *Medical Act 1920* of Tasmania, known as the *Ratten Doubt Revocation Act 1920*.

In the introduction to this book, Dr Hodgson refers to Tasmania as 'a small State with no secrets'. The subject of this biography, Dr Ratten, had many secrets. The facts of his medical 'qualification', his turbulent medico-legal confrontations with professional bodies, his disgrace for race fixing and his disqualification for life by the Tasmanian Turf Club — all are but some of the secrets described in this important biography.

The intriguing story told in this book is one of relatively few professional biographies published to critically record the life and work of an Australian doctor. Of the hundreds of thousands of doctors who have lived and worked in Australia, there are relatively few professional accounts of their lives. This work is a datum study in objectivity. Just as he has brought wisdom and integrity to his many leadership roles in medical practice, so too has the author treated his complex subject with the integrity and objectivity of the professional historian. I commend this book to all with an interest in societal history and to those with specific interests in the history of medicine and the law in Australia.

— *Major General Professor John Pearn AO RFD MD FRACP*
2025

Contents

About the Author 1

Introduction 3

The Dispute 6

Background to the Dispute 9

Resolution of the Dispute 1917-1920 15

The Ratten Family 22

    Arthur Ratten 24

    John Richard Ratten 26

The Early Years 28

Ratten the Dentist 36

American Medical Education 41

Harvey Medical College 43

Sheffield 47

Ratten's Military Career 53

Resolution of the Dispute 1920-1930 59

Private Hospitals in Hobart 62

Resolution of the Dispute 1930-1936 64

Father O'Donnell 68

The Qualities of a Surgeon 71

Ratten's surgical training 74

Ratten's Ability as a Surgeon 76

The Royal Australasian College of Surgeons 87

Ratten as a Person 90

Ratten on the Turf 101

Frauds, Quacks and Impostors 105

Interesting Cases 112

Could it happen again? 116

The Last Years 123

The Final Word 126

Appendix 131

    The Evolution of Healthcare and Healthcare Providers

A note on sources 135

Acknowledgments

I wish to thank the following organisations that have assisted me in one way or another in this project and the following individuals who have listened, commented and advised.

ORGANISATIONS

Archives Tasmania • Australian Society of Anaesthetists
Bland District Historical Society • Brisbane City Council
Dental Board NSW • Dental Board Queensland
Maritime Museum of Tasmania
Medical Board of South Australia
Medical Board of Tasmania
Neurosurgical Society of Australasia Museum
Port Fairy Historical Society
Royal Australasian College of Surgeons
Royal Hobart Hospital Nurses Museum

INDIVIDUALS

Mrs Annette McLean Aherne • Mrs Gillian Allen
Mr Fred Baker • Mrs Rosamond Barber
Mrs Janet Fullerton • Mrs Margie Hodgson
Mr John Lucas • Mrs Amy McGrath • Dr John Morris AO
Dr Andrew Mulcahy • Prof W G Rimmer
Professor Donald Simpson • Dr Philip Thomson
Mrs Judy Tierney OAM • Mrs Barbara Valentine

A note on illustrations

Most images in this book are from the author's collection and several have been digitally repaired and rendered into colour to enhance their effect. Such colour may not be entirely historically accurate but the author believes that it gives new life to old images.

About the Author

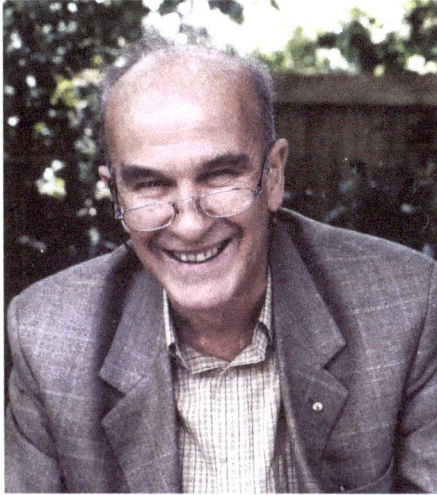

MICHAEL HODGSON AM was born in St Andrews, Scotland in 1941. He migrated to Tasmania with his family in 1947, was educated at the Hobart Technical High School and the University of Queensland, graduating in medicine in 1965.

He trained as an anaesthetist at the Royal Hobart Hospital and the Royal Infirmary, Edinburgh. His career as a specialist anaesthetist has been spent in Hobart.

His interests have been in medical politics, medical administration and medical history, rowing, gardening and long-distance walking, including the Camino.

At State level he has been President of the Australian Medical Association. He was appointed by the Government to the Medical Council of Tasmania in 1982 and became its President in 2000, resigning in 2009 just before the Medical Council was taken over by the new national body, the Australian Health Practitioners Regulation Agency (Ahpra).

He was elected by the medical staff as its member on the Royal Hobart Hospital Board in 1979 and served until the Board became the new Southern Regional Hospitals Board in 1995, when most of the Board were not reappointed.

Nationally, he has been President of the Australian and New Zealand College of Anaesthetists, the Australian Society of Anaesthetists and the Australian Council on Health Care Standards, and has served on the Federal Executive of the Australian Medical Association.

He has been awarded Fellowship of the Australian Medical Association, received the President's award of the Australian Society of Anaesthetists and life membership of the Australian Council on Health Care Standards. He became a Member of the Order of Australia in 1999.

This is his first book.

Introduction

IT WAS 3rd January 1963 and I had just completed my fourth year as a medical student at the University of Queensland. I was working at the Royal Hobart Hospital as a male nurse during my summer vacation, which was possible in those days.

That day, all the nurses who were able to safely leave their patients were instructed to line the balconies at the front of the Hospital when the cortege of an important doctor passed down Liverpool Street on its way to Cornelian Bay Cemetery. I joined them. I learned that the important doctor was (Dr) Victor Richard Ratten.

I had not heard of Ratten until then but I was to learn a lot about him over the next few years — not openly but by way of snide comments from doctors criticising him and from patients who would swear by him. Who was he? Who was this doctor who was so respected by the hospital that he was recognised in this way?

I discovered that one of the principal things so much discussed about Ratten was the question of the validity of his medical qualification.

Ratten had been registered as a medical practitioner by the Court of Medical Examiners in 1907. This was the Government-appointed body responsible for registering medical practitioners in the State under the Medical Act.

On 28th January 1985 I got a phone call from my wife Margie while I was at work. She was at an auction in 'Warinilla', 491 Sandy Bay Road, the home of the recently deceased William Richard ('Barney') Ratten, Victor Ratten's second son.

The auction first involved the contents of the house and then the house itself. Margie told me that Lot 252 was 'Wine store, including wines and pantry,' and asked if I was interested. With no other details available, all I could say was 'If it's going for a song, get it.'

Later that day Margie called again to say that she and her friend Karen Duffy had been successful in their bidding, and asked if I would meet them after work to collect the purchase, which I did.

They had paid $200 and I was not impressed — the lot included old leather boots, framed pictures of no significance, photos that meant nothing to me, several cartons of old red wine of dubious quality and a bottle of French brandy.

While I was taking a load out to my car I looked back and saw Margie holding a cardboard cylinder from which she extracted a rolled paper. Puzzled, I stood transfixed until I saw the excitement on her face.

She had found the long-lost medical diploma of Victor Richard Ratten.

Ratten gained notoriety in Tasmania in 1917. Tasmanian doctors who were members of the British Medical Association (BMA) threatened to withdraw their services from the Hobart General Hospital over an industrial matter. Ratten was not a member of the BMA.

The Government called the BMA's bluff and appointed Ratten surgeon superintendent at the hospital. He was, in today's terminology, a scab. It was an explosive situation. What followed influenced medical practice in Tasmania for decades.

It could only happen in Tasmania — the state with a small population where everyone knows everyone, where patronage is rife and there are no secrets. Put into the mix an intelligent, egotistical, opportunist individual who has, on paper anyway, a medical qualification and a government that wants to teach the BMA a lesson and keep Ratten's services and you have a formula for intrigue, political manoeuvering, self-aggrandisement and opportunities for corruption.

The BMA pursued Ratten. His medical qualification was from the Harvey Medical College in Chicago, Illinois, America and dated 1907 — but the College ceased to exist in 1905.

The Government established a Royal Commission which determined that Ratten's qualification was genuine. By this time the Court of Medical

Examiners had changed to the Medical Council of Tasmania by legislation. The Medical Council investigated Ratten's qualification further. The Government dismissed the members of the Medical Council once and changed the Medical Act three times in an endeavour to prevent the Medical Council from investigating Ratten and possibly deregistering him.

The Government introduced the statute of limitations into the Medical Act, which prevented the Medical Council investigating further. BMA doctors did not return to the Hobart General Hospital until 1930 and Ratten remained Surgeon Superintendent until 1936.

I became fascinated with the whole story of Ratten and read widely, but answers to many questions remained elusive. What was the real story behind Ratten's medical qualification? How good a surgeon was he? And why did the dispute go on for so long?

I gave many talks to medical and community groups on what I knew of Ratten, and people would give me facts and stories. I was often urged to write a book about him.

It has taken me nearly forty years to get to this stage, but the passage of time has allowed me to continue amassing facts and opinions, and my views have matured as I digested all the information and developed a better understanding of events.

In this book I have tried to explain how the dispute arose and how someone without medical qualifications could provide a good surgical service to the community over a professional lifetime. I have tried to get things in context and tried not to judge by today's standards, without taking sides or unfairly criticising the man.

The Dispute

EARLY in 1917 the annual general meeting of the Tasmanian Branch of the British Medical Association unanimously passed this resolution:

'That inasmuch as the Premier has refused to give the British Medical Association (BMA) Tasmanian Branch a definitive assurance that rich and well-to-do patients will not be admitted into State-aided hospitals, the Association has decided that unless the assurance is given by the Premier by 1 March 1917 that such practice will cease, it will instruct all its members to resign forthwith from the honorary staff of such hospitals'.

Confused negotiations followed but agreement could not be reached and all the honorary staff at all State-aided hospitals in Tasmania resigned. A conference was held on 11th April 1917 involving Premier Walter Lee, representatives of the Hospital Board and Drs G H Hogg, G E Clemons, D H E Lines for the BMA and Arthur E Hayward as honorary secretary of the BMA. No solution was found but the resignations were postponed for a week. At its meeting on 16th April 1917 the Hospital Board resolved to continue the existing practice of not admitting wealthy patients to the Hospital and asked the honorary staff to withdraw their resignations.

At its next meeting on 23rd April the Board considered the BMA response, which thanked the Board for its resolution expressing approval of the principle for which the Association was contending and said its members would continue their duties until 28th April if the Premier confirmed a new government policy on the admission of well-to-do patients.

The BMA went on to say that the resignations would take effect immediately if government policy remained unchanged but would be withdrawn if the policy was changed. Resignations would take effect on 28th April if there was no decision by then. The BMA added that it understood that all emergency cases would always be eligible for admission.

The Board urged the BMA not to proceed with the resignations in the interests of the large number of patients in the Hospital. It described it as a drastic step

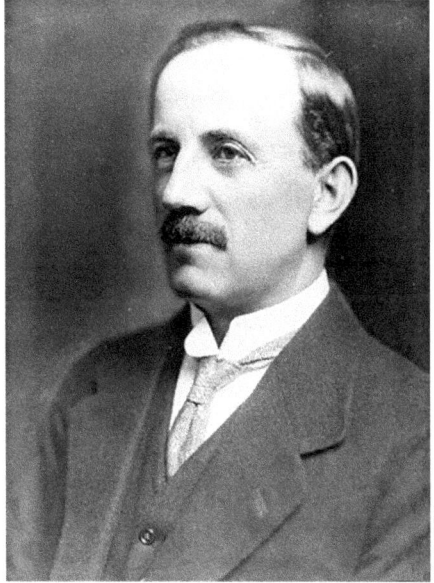

Premier Walter Lee

and suggested it would be best to await the Premier's response because the Board could not comply with the request. The Premier had promised to deal quickly with the Hospital Bill, which would be submitted to the Board and the BMA before going to Parliament; the Bill would define administrative arrangements for medical staffing. On 28th April the BMA wrote again to the Board, saying that the resignations must now take effect and reiterated that honoraries would attend to emergency cases when requested by the resident staff.

The Board accepted the resignations at its meeting on 30th April and by 4th May the hospital was without resident staff when the last two left. Dr T H Goddard, the house surgeon, resigned and Dr J H McCutcheon was called up for military duty. The hospital then had no medical assistance.

The BMA was obviously concerned about the situation because it wrote to the Hospital again on 7th May, asking whether the Board would accept the offer of the honorary staff to assist the house surgeon when requested.

The dispute came to an end on 14th May 1917 when the Government unexpectedly, and as a great shock to the BMA, announced that it had

— 7 —

appointed Victor Richard Ratten as surgeon superintendent, Dr E T MacGowan as visiting surgeon and Dr E L Crowther as anaesthetist at the Hospital. On 16th May the secretary of the Board wrote to the BMA: 'I am directed to inform you that arrangements have been made to carry out the professional work of the Institution.'

Doctors Crowther and MacGowan did not have honorary positions at the time; both were members of the BMA and both resigned their memberships. They were appointed to the Medical Council of Tasmania.

Ratten was to be paid a salary of £750 a year plus living quarters, light and fuel and was allowed to take part in consultations. MacGowan was paid £400, had no quarters and was allowed the right of private practice. Crowther was paid an honorarium of £200.

Note: Honorary Staff (Honoraries).

There were a limited number in each public hospital. Medical practitioners applied, their names went before the current honoraries in the hospital and those selected were appointed by the hospital board. They were not paid, and they were not allowed to charge patients under their care in the hospital.

Background to the Dispute

THE DISPUTE involved three parties: the BMA, the Tasmanian Government and Ratten, at a time when the medical profession was not well organised. The event said to have started it arose in 1917 when a well-to-do patient from Hobart went to Launceston to be operated on by Dr Sweetnam, the surgeon superintendent at the Launceston General Hospital.

Mr H M Wright, a long-serving secretary at the Hobart General Hospital, believed that the trouble started when the reputedly very wealthy Miss Brock broke her leg horse riding and went to the Launceston General Hospital for treatment because there she could be under the personal care of surgeon superintendent Dr H W Sweetnam. Many of the very capable doctors — W W Giblin, D H E Lines, Campbell, W E L H Crowther and others — were on active service and of those who did not enlist Sweetman was by far the most capable surgeon in Tasmania. As well, transportation to Melbourne was slow and infrequent.

Surgeons in the south felt that Launceston surgeons had cause for complaint; they joined forces and resolved that the issue was one for the BMA.

Earlier, Dr John Ramsay (later Sir John Ramsay — the first surgeon in Australia to be knighted) was surgeon superintendent at the Launceston General Hospital from 1898 to 1912 and was considered a good surgeon. He also ran a large private practice, consulting and operating at the local Waratah Hospital. This annoyed local doctors who considered it unfair competition in that they worked as honoraries at the Hospital.

The Government responded by enacting the Launceston General Hospital Act 1910 which specifically forbade doctors at the Hospital engaging in private practice outside the hospital. Dr Ramsay resigned in 1912 and was replaced by Dr Sweetnam.

In 1887 Dr Smart chaired a small committee of medical practitioners in Hobart with the aim of establishing a branch of the BMA in Tasmania, but without success. In 1896 Sir James Agnew was largely responsible for the establishment in the Royal Society of Medicine of a Medical Section which considered the educational and professional interests of medical practitioners. In 1897 practitioners in northern Tasmania organised themselves as a subdivision of the Victorian Branch of the BMA and one of its early actions was to ask the Board of the Launceston General Hospital to reduce the powers of the surgeon superintendent and subsequently a Select Committee of Inquiry removed the right of the surgeon superintendent to conduct private practice. In February 1902, at the Sixth Session of the Intercolonial Medical Congress of Australasia held in Hobart, a proposal to establish an Australian Medical Association was not approved but it was agreed that the congress be renamed the Australasian Medical Congress.

The Tasmanian Branch of the BMA was finally established on 22nd July 1911 following a meeting called by Dr Sprott. Ratten was declared ineligible for membership on account of his American qualifications.

As with the Australian Medical Association (AMA) of today, the BMA looked after the professional interests of its members, including industrial matters.

Outside influences now came into play. The BMA in Australia and in other parts of the Empire and the Australian Medical Congress had a policy of excluding well-to-do patients from public hospitals. This was pointed out to the Lee government, but they were unsympathetic. The policy is quite understandable — doctors were working unpaid, yet they were being asked to treat well-to-do patients for nothing, effectively undermining their private practices.

Public hospitals were considered charitable organisations. Money was donated and bequeathed by the public for the care of the sick-poor by honorary medical practitioners. As Dr James Walch put it — under the

Hospitals Act public hospitals were established to treat the sick, the poor and, by implication, not the well-to-do.

The BMA approached Premier Lee to ask that the new legislation should deny admission of well-to-do patients to public hospitals because it was contrary to the purpose of Government general hospitals and negatively affected the interests of the medical profession.

There were long-standing divisions within the medical profession and one of these revolved around the fact that there were those who had honorary positions at the public hospitals and those that did not, and it was regarded as something of a closed shop. When the dispute arose, some doctors would not toe the BMA line and there was a lack of unity. Among other issues which could have led to this situation was the north-south conflict that persists even today. Northern doctors had earlier become a subdivision of the Victorian Branch of the BMA and now with the new Tasmanian branch of the BMA, the president who was elected at the Annual General Meeting rotated between north and south, which could have exacerbated this lack of unity and continuity.

There were some strong personalities within the BMA. Dr Hogg in his Presidential Address in 1914 said:

'A section of the public is (sic) apt to think that our aims are selfish ones. I know of no more unselfish profession than ours: whether it be in our organisations, or our everyday work, in our research, we spend not only money but what is far more valuable than money, brains, bodies and too often our lives in the attempt to lessen the aggregate of disease, suffering and death. If the BMA in addition to playing a great part in this our life's work also does the best to see that the conditions under which we work are fair and just surely the people as well as the state should not forget that the 'labourer is worthy of his hire'.

Other things influenced the thinking of the BMA: the viability of private practice, the standard of American medical qualifications and the consequences of World War I. As well, friendly societies, the forerunners of today's private health insurers, were reluctant to increase the fees of medical practitioners.

The BMA denied membership to medical practitioners with American medical qualifications, even if they were registered in the State.

There was anxiety in the profession about the war, about the current workload with many doctors on active service, protecting the practice of medicine financially and protecting the practices of doctors on active service.

When Ratten arrived in Hobart in 1916 he bought Dr Wolfhagen's practice. This created a stir, and he was viewed with suspicion because there was an understanding that for the duration of the war no practitioner would encroach upon the practice of a doctor who was on active service. A special meeting of the British Medical Corps Association considered Ratten's arrival, but no action was taken because Ratten had bought an existing practice, Dr Wolfhagen's; this was not considered contrary to the understanding since Dr Wolfhagen was retiring because of ill-health.

Medical practitioners were organising themselves and flexing their muscles, but without unity of purpose.

At the time Premier Lee was a Nationalist; there was no formal party system as we know it today. He was from the same electorate as Ratten, they were friends and he was likely Ratten's ally in the dispute.

It has been said over the years that it was Labor Premiers who conspired to defeat the BMA and appoint Ratten. This is not borne out by facts because between 1907, when Ratten appeared on the scene, and 1917 when the dispute occurred, the Premiers were: John Evans (Anti Socialist), Sir Elliot Lewis (Liberal), John Earle (Labor), Albert Solomon (Commonwealth Liberal) and Walter Lee (Commonwealth Liberal/Nationalist). Further, in the period after Ratten's 1917 appointment and his resignation in 1936, the Nationalists were in power for twelve years and Labor for seven.

The Medical Act 1908 changed the Court of Medical Examiners to the Medical Council of Tasmania. Importantly, it clarified which qualifications were acceptable for registration in Tasmania and barred American qualifications.

At the time there were four practitioners registered with American qualifications and the Medical Council of Tasmania put them on a separate list at the end of the publicly available register of medical practitioners. Ratten said that he would fight as hard and for as long as needed to have this decision reversed and American medical qualifications fully recognised again.

The administration of public hospitals had been an issue for government for some time and in 1878, 1882 and 1900 specific legislation was passed regulating both the Launceston General Hospital and the Hobart General Hospital.

In 1914, Dr McClintock, the Chief Medical Officer for Tasmania, was appointed a sole Royal Commissioner to inquire into the existing unsatisfactory administration of public hospitals in the State. He stated in his report that the Hobart General Hospital was the worst-conducted institution of its class he had ever visited, and that the inbred honorary system of medical staffing encouraged patronage. One of his principal recommendations was that hospitals be taken over by the State — nationalised.

The Government appointed an enlarged Commission to inquire into the Hobart General Hospital and decided to draft a new Hospitals Act.

Notwithstanding the strength of the BMA, the obvious lack of unity within the medical profession must have encouraged the Government in its actions, which with their implicit intent must have concerned the BMA.

Before the dispute, Ratten probably felt threatened. He must have felt aggrieved to be declared ineligible for BMA membership — and his purchase of Dr Wolfhagen's practice in 1916 was being questioned. He certainly would have been worried about his potentially precarious future, so when the Government offered him the position of surgeon superintendent he readily accepted because it made him more secure. He kept a low profile and did not make himself a target at the time.

So behind the dispute we see an uncompromising BMA, a determined Government and an opportunistic Ratten.

Dr Goddard was interviewed in 1960 and added to the story about events in 1917. He said that in the two-and-a-half years before Ratten's appointment he had been administratively medical superintendent at the hospital, with surgical services provided by honoraries. There was no problem with well-to-do patients being admitted to the hospital and this was supported by the hospital board. In Launceston there was a salaried full-time surgeon superintendent. There was a problem with well-to-do patients in that hospital.

When the BMA doctors resigned from the Hobart General Hospital the staffing situation was not as dramatic as it seemed. Dr Goddard was approached by the Premier and the chairman of the hospital board with the request that he remain as medical superintendent, but as this virtually meant his withdrawal from the BMA and as he was quite a young man at the beginning of his medical life, he could not accept this and resigned.

He told the board that he would stay at the hospital long enough for new medical officers to get to know the patients and he continued giving anaesthetics for Ratten until the new regime had settled in.

As stated by Rebekah McWhirter: 'Social conflict takes the form of competition for resources between rival interest groups', and 'In a conflict between the interests of medical practitioners and the interests of state aided hospitals one had to lose'.

Resolution of the Dispute
1917-1920

OVER THE next three years the BMA, the Government and the Medical Council of Tasmania made a series of moves with Ratten central to them all. It was a real chess game which the Government and Ratten ultimately won.

The BMA attacked the man, the Government protected the man.

Prior to his appointment as surgeon superintendent Ratten was probably already feeling persecuted. The Government had legislated that American medical graduates were no longer eligible for registration as a medical practitioner in Tasmania. The BMA had declared Ratten ineligible for membership of their Association based on his American medical qualification.

The Australian Medical Corps Association, which had a policy of protecting the practices of members serving with the Armed Forces, had held a special meeting to consider the propriety of Ratten's taking over Dr Wolfhagen's practice in Hobart, but this was accepted since Dr Wolfhagen was retiring due to ill health.

The BMA was now asking questions about irregularities in Ratten's medical qualification and about Ratten having been warned off the Newnham Racing Club by the stewards for allegedly fixing races.

The BMA did not want to be seen as the body making the complaints about Ratten and requested the Medical Council to investigate and, if appropriate, prosecute. This was and still is the accepted way for a complaint against a medical practitioner to be made and considered.

It is interesting to follow the Government's moves.

When the BMA started to accuse Ratten of obtaining his medical qualification by fraud, the Medical Council decided to ask the four registered medical practitioners with American medical qualifications to produce their diplomas and supply detail of their courses of study.

The Premier challenged the validity of the Medical Council's action and Ratten assured the Premier that the accusations were unfounded and asked for a public inquiry to be set up to clear his name. The Premier agreed.

A Royal Commission headed by Justice Norman K Ewing first sat on 16th November 1918. Justice Ewing determined that the Harvey Medical College existed in 1907 and that Ratten had received his diploma from the College. Ratten was represented by Mr M W Hodgman.

The Commissioner sent a cable to the Attorney General of Illinois asking whether the Harvey Medical College legally existed on 8th March 1907 and received no reply.

He followed this up with a cable to Dr French, President of the Board of Directors of the Harvey Medical College, and asked him if he issued the diploma to Ratten in March 1907 and what were the relations between Harvey Medical College and Harvey-Jenner College.

French replied: 'Diploma issued Victor Richard Ratten March 1907 by me and others on behalf Harvey no connection with Harvey-Jenner College. W G French'.

The Commissioner had further communications from the American Medical Association that Ratten was not a student or graduate from official lists of the Harvey Medical College and from an attorney in Chicago that the Harvey Medical College was a duly chartered institution in1907.

The Commissioner at this stage stated that strictly speaking there was no evidence before him which would have been accepted by a court of law.

He then questioned Ratten about where the College was, about the number of lectures he received and who delivered them. He went on to say that this information from Ratten was really the only sworn testimony of real value before him, but taking this into account, the cables he received from Illinois, submissions by the parties and his reading of the American Medical Journal, he was prepared to make these findings:

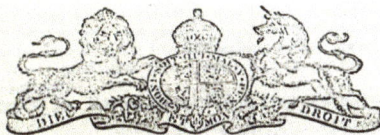

(No. 55.)

1918.

PARLIAMENT OF TASMANIA.

CHARGES MADE BY EDWARD BRETTING- HAM MOORE AGAINST VICTOR RICHARD RATTEN:

REPORT OF ROYAL COMMISSION.

Ordered by the House of Assembly to be printed, December 17, 1918

[Estimated cost of printing (250)—£2 10s.]

REPORT.

To His Excellency SIR FRANCIS ALEXANDER NEWDIGATE NEWDEGATE, Knight Commander of the Most Distinguished Order of Saint Michael and Saint George, Governor in and over the State of Tasmania and its Dependencies, in the Commonwealth of Australia.

MAY IT PLEASE YOUR EXCELLENCY :

I, the Commissioner appointed by His Majesty's Commission, dated the 9th of November, 1918, having inquired into the matters set forth therein, have the honour to submit to Your Excellency my Report.

The Commission opened at The Supreme Court House, Hobart, on the 15th day of November, 1918, and there were four subsequent sittings.

Prior to the sitting of the Commission I received an intimation from Dr. D. H. Harvey, President of the Tasmanian Branch of the British Medical Association, that for reasons which had been stated in a letter to the Honourable the Premier, the British Medical Association did not intend to take any part in the inquiry.

Mr. F. Lodge applied for leave to appear on behalf of the Medical Council of Tasmania, which was granted. Mr. M. W. Hodgman applied for leave to appear for Dr. Ratten, and this also was granted.

The British Medical Association tendered no evidence in support of the charges, but I caused Dr. Brettingham-Moore to appear before me, and although he stated that he still had reason to believe he was right in persisting in the charges

(1) That the Harvey Medical College, Chicago, in the State of Illinois, in the United States of America, did exist in the year 1907.

(2) That the diploma, which the said Victor Richard Ratten produced in

— 17 —

Tasmania in the year 1907, and by which he received registration as a legally qualified medical practitioner, was granted to him by the said Harvey Medical College.

Ratten's responses to questions were not very enlightening:

Your name is Victor Richard Ratten?

Yes.

You are a medical practitioner practising in Hobart?

Yes.

At present you are surgeon-superintendent at the Hobart General Hospital?

Yes.

You recognise the certificate I hold in my hand?

Yes.

Was that certificate issued to you?

Yes.

By the Harvey Medical College?

Yes.

Was it then an existing institution to your knowledge?

Yes.

The BMA did not give evidence at the Royal Commission because it believed the terms of reference were too narrow. As is often said — 'Never hold an inquiry unless you know what the answer is going to be,' and 'The answer you get depends on the questions you ask'.

Ratten was a friend of Justice Ewing.

The Government's next move was to change the Medical Act in 1918 to control the activities of the Medical Council and to allow for certain American medical qualifications to be recognised if the person was registered in the American state in which the diploma was obtained. This did not help Ratten because he was not registered in the state in which he had received his diploma. The Government also appointed to the Medical Council a majority of members who were known to be sympathetic to Ratten and its cause.

This did not change the approach of the Medical Council. Medical Acts have a clause that if a complaint is received it must be considered; it is a legal requirement and if the BMA made a complaint it had to be considered.

The BMA continued to investigate Ratten and obtained evidence that the Ratten diploma was forged by William French, one of the signatories to his diploma. This evidence had been obtained by Andrew Inglis Clark, a member of the Tasmanian Bar, who had been requested by the BMA to include a visit to Chicago whilst returning from the First World War.

The BMA medical practitioners would not consult with Ratten and were effectively isolating him medically. The BMA inserted notices in the *Medical Journal of Australia* requesting that medical practitioners wanting to apply for medical position in Tasmanian public hospitals communicate with the BMA first.

The Medical Council continued investigating.

The Government changed the Medical Act again and every change was specifically aimed at overcoming difficulties that could make it harder for Ratten to retain registration.

Now:

- Only a Supreme Court judge could authorise the deregistration of a doctor on the grounds of fraud;
- The Court or Judge could authorise the examination of witnesses at any place;
- It became an offence to refuse to consult with another medical practitioner and the practitioner seeking the advice was legally liable for the fee;
- It became an offence to prevent in any way any person applying for a position in any State-aided hospital; and
- American qualifications were to be recognised if they were registered in one of the States of the United States of America.

Medical Appointments.

IMPORTANT NOTICE.

Medical practitioners are requested not to apply for any appointment referred to in the following table, without having first communicated with the Honorary Secretary of the Branch named in the first column, or with the Medical Secretary of the British Medical Association, 429 Strand, London, W.C.

Branch.	APPOINTMENTS.
VICTORIA. (Hon. Sec., Medical Society Hall, East Melbourne.)	All Friendly Society Lodges, Institutes, Medical Dispensaries and other Contract Practice. Australian Prudential Association Proprietary, Limited. Mutual National Provident Club. National Provident Association.
QUEENSLAND. (Hon. Sec., B.M.A. Building, Adelaide Street, Brisbane.)	Australian Natives' Association. Brisbane United Friendly Society Institute. Cloncurry Hospital.
TASMANIA. (Hon. Sec., Macquarie Street, Hobart.)	Medical Officers in all State-aided Hospitals in Tasmania.

AUTHOR'S COLLECTION

The Medical Council believed they were right and by May 1920 they felt that they had enough evidence to charge Ratten with obtaining his medical registration by fraud. This required them to take the matter to the Supreme Court because of the recent changes to the Medical Act. Only a Supreme Court Judge could authorise the deregistration of a doctor on the grounds of fraud.

Surprisingly, the Government agreed to indemnify the Medical Council for its costs in the proceedings and to indemnify Ratten if he was successful in defending himself.

The case never got off the ground.

The Chief Justice hearing the case, Sir Herbert Nichols, refused to allow evidence taken on oath in America to be presented to the Court, so the Medical Council could not proceed. Recent changes to the Medical Act had said 'The court or judge could authorise the examination of witnesses at any place'.

The Chief Justice said that this was a case in which the jury should see and hear witnesses. Moreover, the defendant should be present when witnesses were being examined.

The Law Society publicly disagreed with this ruling.

The Medical Council considered appealing to the High Court, having received advice from its lawyers that it would probably, on appeal, reverse the decision of the Chief Justice. The Government refused to pay the Council's expenses.

The final move came with the passing of an act to further amend the Medical Act 1918, known as the Medical Act 1920 or the Ratten Doubt Revocation Act. This act invoked the statute of limitations, providing that the offence which is the basis for an application to deregister a medical practitioner on the grounds of fraud must have been committed in the previous seven years. This was 1920 and Ratten was originally registered in 1907.

Albert Ogilvie drafted this Act, which passed both Houses of Parliament — the House of Assembly and the Legislative Council — in one day!

This was the coup de grâce to the BMA and it made Ratten's position secure.

At the time of writing there have been sixteen instances where Doubts Removal Bills have been put before the Tasmanian Parliament and only one was not passed. All were to correct illegal situations but none involved significant events. Dr Frank Madill, a member of the House of Assembly, in his book *Why Politics Doctor* recounts a situation in which his medical practice, the Ravenswood Health Centre, had a contract with the Health Department, which was illegal for a parliamentarian. The amount in question was $71.93. When he put the situation before the Premier the conversation went:

'I see,' said Robin (Gray), 'Don't worry, Frankie (Madill), we'll just have to put through a Doubts Removal Bill'.

'I looked at him in disbelief. Could it really be as simple and easy as that?' said Dr Madill.

The Ratten Family

VICTOR RICHARD RATTEN, the eldest of six children, was born on 12 December 1878 in Kew, Victoria, to George William Ratten (1859-1929), a teacher, and Eliza Annie Ratten (née Gordon). His family can be traced back to Thomas Ratten and his wife Harriet (née Mummery) of Kent, England who also had six children and arrived in Victoria in January 1842 on the barque *Sarah*. Three other children were listed on Thomas Ratten's death certificate.

One of the children, Richard (1832-1879), married Fanny Bird and had ten children; the eldest boy, George William, was Victor Richard Ratten's father. George was the second child. Fanny Bird had been baptised in Barrington, Cambridgeshire and they named their family home 'Barrington' when they came to Victoria. Interestingly, Victor Richard Ratten's marriage certificate mistakenly indicates that he was born in Barrington, England.

Another of Richard Ratten's sons was Arthur Ratten (1860-1943), who obtained a Bachelor of Arts degree from the University of Melbourne, and some years later obtained an MA, PhD and MD from Boston in America —but more of that later.

Two of his four children should be noted — Rosamond (Bartie), the author of *The Pioneer Rattens of Two Continents* and Cecil Aurelius, who early in his career worked as a signalman for the South Australian Railways.

George Ratten's second son was Frederick William Ratten, who married Ella Mary Field, the daughter of a family with large property interests in Tasmania. They spent much of their married life in Queensland.

On 29th October 1907 Victor Richard married Violet (Blanche) Cecily Greaves, daughter of an Irish hotelkeeper in Brisbane. They had two children, Jack (John) Richard, born on 14th November 1909 and William Richard, born on 14th November 1911.

William Richard Ratten was a businessman in Hobart; he died in 1984. John Richard Ratten was an engineer and inspector of mines in North Queensland prior to World War II. During the war he was a Wing Commander and led a Spitfire squadron in England. He died on 27th February 1945 aged 35.

Victor Ratten died in Hobart on 30th December 1962.

Arthur Ratten

ARTHUR was Ratten's uncle and was born in Kew, Victoria in 1860. He graduated with a Bachelor of Arts (BA) from Melbourne University in 1882.

He had four children, including Cecil Aurelius who became a railwayman in South Australia and Rosamond (Barber) who later wrote a book: *The Pioneer Rattens of two continents, Australia and North America.*

Arthur established Oriel College for boys in Kew, an advertisement stating:

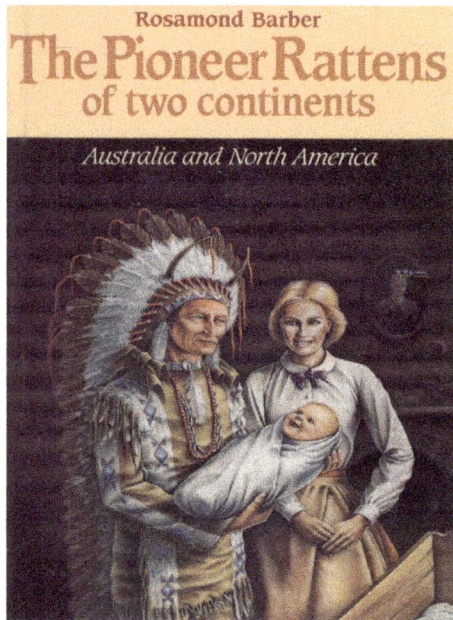

Rosamond Barber
The Pioneer Rattens
of two continents
Australia and North America

'Oriel College, Kew Heights, Glenferrie Road. Headmaster: Arthur Ratten BA (Melb. 1882). Formerly Senior (Resident) Master, Scotch College, Hobart, and Hurstville College, NSW. Visiting Matriculation Master, Melbourne College, and nearly 20 years continuous experience, Arts, Matric., Public Service, Pharmacy and evening classes and Private Tuition orally or by post. Third term July 15th'.'

It was for a time a flourishing concern, but the troubled economy of the times meant that many patrons were unable to pay the fees and a decision had to be made about the future of the College. Arthur decided he would be a doctor. He went to Boston, Massachusetts, and gained a Doctor of Philosophy in 1898, a Master of Arts in 1899 and a Doctor of Medicine (MD) in 1900, working in the Homeopathic Dispensary.

After further experience in America he returned to Melbourne and became a very successful medical practitioner, dying in 1943.

Perhaps Arthur's success in obtaining medical qualifications influenced Victor Ratten to do likewise.

John Richard Ratten

RATTEN'S first son, christened Jack but known as John, was born in Sheffield, Tasmania, on 13th November 1909. He was educated at Launceston Church Grammar School and graduated as a mining engineer at the Mount Lyell School of Mines, part of the University of Tasmania. He was married to Barbara Hurst and had two children, John Hugill Greaves and Gillian.

At the time of his enlistment in the Royal Australian Air Force on 31st January 1941 he was a government mining inspector in North Queensland.

He became a Squadron Leader in the Royal Air Force and was awarded the Distinguished Flying Cross (DFC) on 15th June 1943, his citation reading; 'Squadron Leader Ratten has completed a large number of sorties and has led the squadron and often the wing with great skill. This officer has rendered excellent service, setting a most praiseworthy example. He has destroyed one and shared in the destruction of another enemy aircraft'.

His death has been attributed in various publications to a car accident, active service and tuberculosis.

The RAF explained 'It was on flying duties that John first sustained an injury to his ear as a result of which he later underwent a mastoid operation. In consequence of this operation his general health and physical condition became very much lowered, and he contracted a tubercular infection in both lungs'. He died in England on 27th February 1945 aged 35 years.

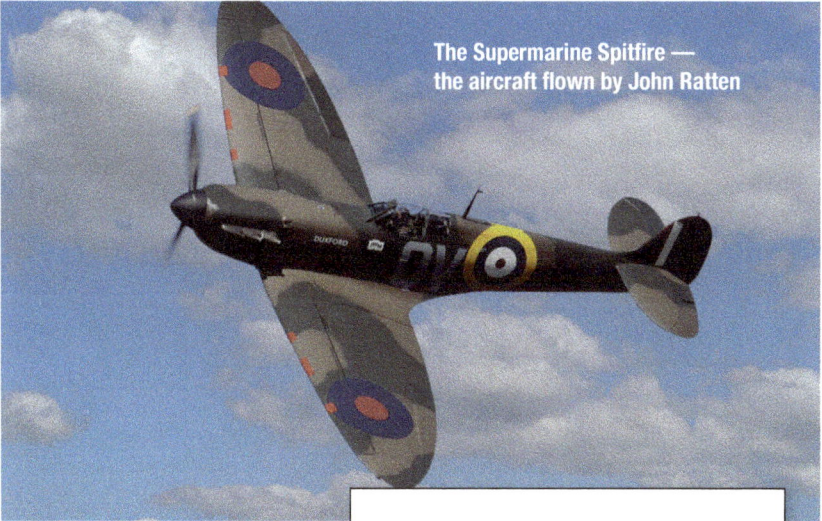

The Supermarine Spitfire — the aircraft flown by John Ratten

WIKIPEDIA

During the war the return to Australia of the remains or ashes of members of the Royal Australian Air Force who died overseas whilst on active service was prohibited by the Australian Government.

John Ratten's ashes were therefore interred at the Brighton Downs Crematorium.

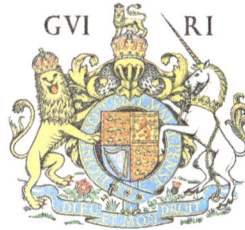

GVI RI

This scroll commemorates
Wing Commander J. R. Ratten, D.F.C.
Royal Australian Air Force
held in honour as one who
served King and Country in
the world war of 1939-1945
and gave his life to save
mankind from tyranny. May
his sacrifice help to bring
the peace and freedom for
which he died.

AUTHOR'S COLLECTION

The Early Years

RELATIVELY little is known about Ratten's early years and I have done the best I can by following his father's movements. These were uncertain times, particularly during the great depression in the 1890s.

George Ratten established a college in Port Fairy in Victoria in a building which was originally the Stag Hotel. The Borough rent book shows he paid rates in the years 1890 to 1893-4, the next rate book is missing and there is no record in the book for 1896, so probably the College opened in the early 1890s and closed some time in 1894 or 1895. The premises were built in 1847 and were known as Seacombe House. Today it is a guesthouse and has not been much altered.

Unfortunately, no school rolls for Port Fairy College seem to be in the public record. In 1936 there might have been a reunion of Port Fairy College students because in the *Age* newspaper of 30th May there appears this reminiscence:

'In the early 90's Mr Ratten had a school at Port Fairy, a feature of which was the cadet corps, with uniforms, Franchi rifles, drums and bugles. The cadets had a fine time; trips to various towns, Hamilton, Portland etc and engaging in shooting and other competitions.

'Who remembers the fight after hours between Vic Ratten and Les Earle that took place in the stable at the back of the school? Posy Howell was door man, and the sequel was enacted next day when Mr Ratten called all scholars into the big room and producing his green hide thong whip proceeded to deal with the fighters'.

Another reference to the College building is a description by a recent

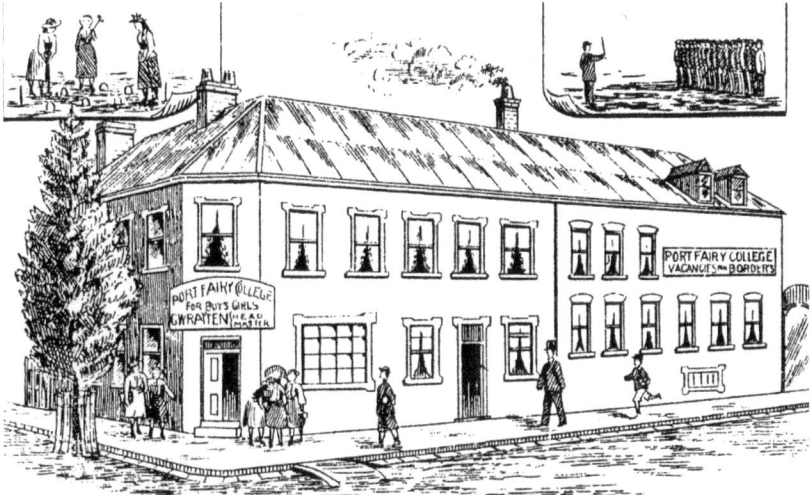

PORT FAIRY COLLEGE (Boys and Girls). G. W. Ratten, Head Master.
Unqualified Success in all kinds of Examinations. Ninety-five per cent. Passes obtained.
Over 100 pupils have already passed. Commercial Classes a Speciality. All the Educational
Advantages combined with the Pleasures of the Seaside—Bathing, Shelling, Beaches, &c.
Perfect Climate. The Sanatorium of Victoria. Delicate Pupils especially cared for.

arrival from England in the mid 1850s: 'Strange it is to look through the range of little rooms, with windows deep in the walls and ceilings sloping downwards and in the whole great building, only three fireplaces.

By 1895 Ratten was aged 17 years and had possibly left school. Records of his movements are somewhat sketchy, but it is reasonably safe to assume that he remained with the family and his father's employment gives clues to where he was and what he was doing.

In 1895 George opened a private college in Parkes, NSW, which failed. In 1897 he opened Lachlan College in Forbes, NSW. Whether Victor attended these Colleges is unknown, but he must have sought employment about then because in June 1898 he resigned from a position at the Union Bank in Forbes.

On 11th June 1898 it was reported that he was departing on a bicycle tour of the world, but Victor and his friend did not get out of Sydney. Was it a case of no money, or was his teacher father telling him to get a career? Did an opportunity arise for him to be apprenticed to a dentist?

Important changes were occurring in the family. His father, who had run colleges in Port Fairy, Parkes and Forbes, was ordained in 1898-1899 and was deacon at the local church in Forbes.

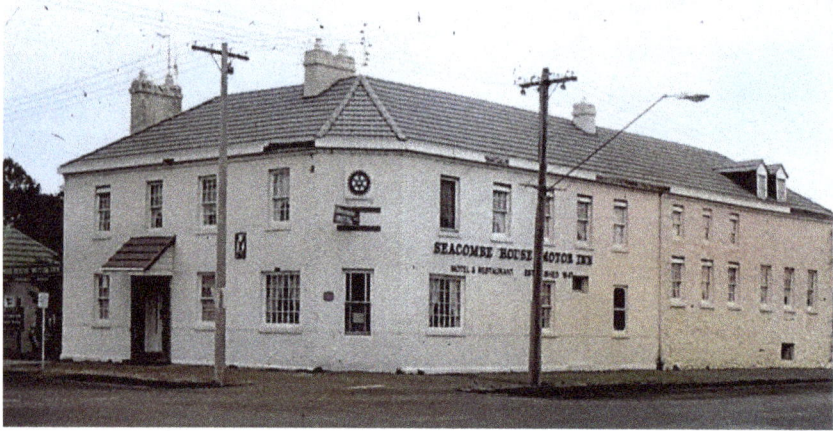

Ratten is said to have been apprenticed to a dentist in Sydney and this could only have been in late 1898-1899. He commenced a dental practice in Wyalong, NSW and registered as a dentist on 1st February 1901 when the Dental Act 1900 was passed. He then moved to Queensland, establishing a dental practice in Queen Street, Brisbane. He registered as a dentist in Queensland on 16th July 1903, but that is a story for later and he was there until at least 1906. His only recorded residence is given as Hotel Cecil, George St, Brisbane. After this his movements are well documented but there are several conflicting statements about them.

He worked for three years as a dental mechanic in Texas, USA. There is no record of this and no time for him to have done that.

He acted as a dresser in the Maryborough Hospital but hospitals with that name in Victoria and Queensland have no record of him. A dresser was the equivalent of a hospital orderly today, but it was also the name of a person apprenticed to a medical practitioner.

He was for three years a medical student in Australia. There is no time for him to have done this and medical schools in existence at the time have no record of him.

He was apprenticed to a dentist in Sydney. This is possible, but again there is no record of this, and it could not have been for very long.

Ratten left Australia on 3rd September 1906 on the passenger ship *Aorangi* to Vancouver, Canada, went by rail to Chicago and obtained a diploma Doctor of Medicine (MD) from the Harvey Medical College,

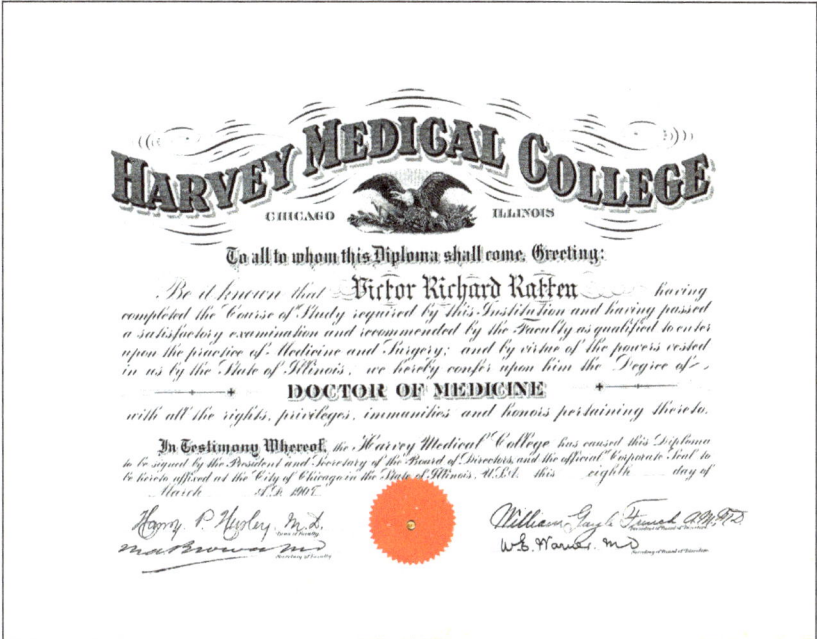

*Ratten's bogus diploma is an impressively large document,
measuring 557 by 430mm*

Chicago, Illinois dated 8 March 1907. He then obtained a licence to practise medicine, surgery and obstetrics in the state of Texas, dated 12th
March 1907. Why did Ratten go to America to get a medical qualification?' The most likely explanation is that he had seen his uncle Arthur
Ratten go to Boston in 1900 and get an MD without too much trouble.
But mind you, he also collected a Master of Arts and Doctor of Philosophy over two years!

Ratten must have been on the way back to Australia before obtaining
his MD and registering in Texas because on 24th February 1907 he is
reported to have been in Liverpool, England and Queenstown in Ireland.
Queenstown, renamed Cobh in 1920 during the Irish war of independ-
ence, was a major port for prisoners being sent to penal colonies including Australia and the most important emigration port for immigrants to
North America. It was the final departure port of the *Titanic* in 1912 and
also of RMS *Lusitania*, sunk by the Germans in1915.

THE STATE OF TEXAS

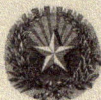

To Whomsoever It May Concern:

The undersigned Board of Medical Examiners, acting for, and by the authority of the State of Texas, under the medical practice law of 1901, having examined

V R Ratten M D

in all the professional subjects required by said law, and having found _him_ proficient therein, do hereby issue to _him_ this

License

to practice Medicine, Surgery and Obstetrics, in the State of Texas.

In testimony whereof we have hereto subscribed our names, and caused the seal of the State to be affixed this _Twelfth_ day of _March_ 1907 _at Dallas Texas_

H B Stillwann M D
SECRETARY

J R Pollock M D
F L Griffith M D
Wm Smith M D
Chas E Johnson M D
W G Thatcher M D

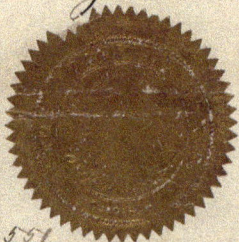

557

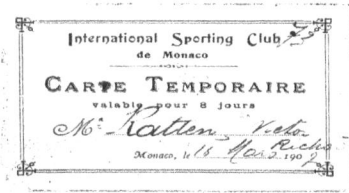
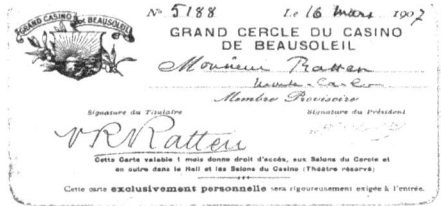
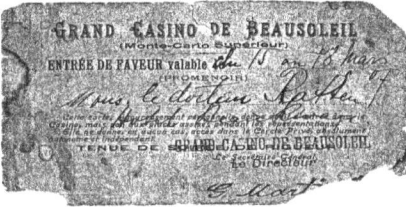
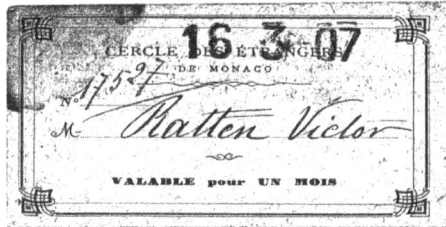

Evidence of a little mis-spent youth?

He is known to have been in Monte Carlo from 16th-18th March 1907 and arrived back in Australia some time before 9th May 1907. He had been away eight months and was 29 years old.

He registered as a medical practitioner in South Australia and Tasmania — the only states in Australia that recognised American Medical qualifications.

Ratten registered in South Australia on 9th May 1907, stating that he had been a dentist in Queensland, Brisbane and Maryborough, before returning to America. He produced his diploma and signed a statutory declaration dated 3rd May 1907, saying that he was the same V R Ratten whose name appears on the diploma and that it had been after at least four years of study. In 1920, as a result of an enquiry from the Medical Council of Tasmania, the South Australian Medical Board Registrar indicated that the only surviving member of the Board that had regis-tered Ratten was the President and replied: 'I presume that Ratten pro-vided some evidence that he could practice in Illinois — at the same time it must be admitted that the Board was occasionally harassed by minis-ters and lawyers and obliged under the threat of mandamus to register such persons — still, neither our President nor I can recall this as being one of such cases'.

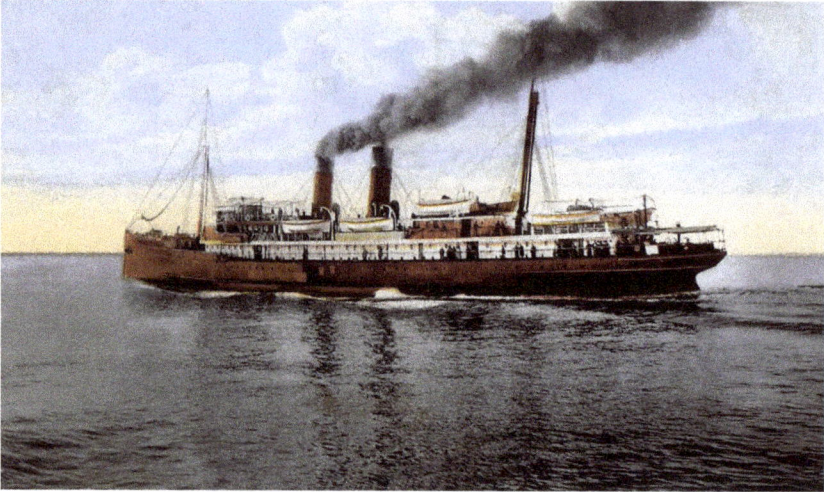

TSS Loongana *crossing Bass Strait 1n 1913*

Ratten did not stay to practise in South Australia but quickly moved to Tasmania on the TSS *Loongana* from Melbourne to Launceston, arriving on 21st May 1907. He registered with the Court of Medical Examiners on the following day. Registration as a medical practitioner required posses-sion of a qualification described in the schedule of the medical act and proof on personal attendance that the document testifying to his quali-fication was obtained after examination by the recognised body in the country in which it was obtained. Ratten obviously satisfied the court of medical examiners at the time.

On 5th June 1907 he is recorded as passing through Wallangarra, Queensland, which is near the border with New South Wales, on the mail train for Brisbane.

By 8th June 1907 he was being interviewed by a journalist about his extensive tour of the world and recounted his interesting experiences. He said that he had spent eight months in Chicago, did a medical course at Chicago University and obtained an MD, adding that he had previously put in four years there. He listed places he had visited including Niagara, New York, London, Paris and Italy, returning via the Suez Canal on a Cunard liner.

He married Blanche Cecily Greaves, daughter of an Irish hotelkeeper in Brisbane, on 29th October 1907 at St Mary's Church, Kangaroo Point. With his new wife he visited Sheffield, Tasmania on 11th January 1908, found that there was an opening for a medical practitioner and decided to settle there. Dr Ed Chisholm was returning to NSW and the other medical practitioner in the town at the time, Dr Davis, was quite elderly and died shortly afterwards. His father was at this time rector at nearby Stanley.

Ratten quickly established himself in the community: he built a residence and a hospital, St Helens Hospital, on adjoining blocks at the corner of Main and Henry Streets and took part in local activities. He purchased a barber shop and billiard saloon, became a Justice of the Peace, and served as Officer of Health for the Kentish Municipality.

It was said that although he was only there for a few short years he left his mark like no other doctor.

He was commissioned as a temporary Captain (Medical Officer) in the 12th battalion, Australian Imperial Forces on 20th August 1914. On 20th October 1914 he sailed on the SS *Geelong*, the first ship to carry troops of the Expeditionary Force to World War I.

Following his return to Tasmania his appointment was terminated on 13th March 1915 and he soon decided to leave Sheffield and move to Hobart, where he bought Dr Wolfhagen's practice.

In early 1917 a dispute arose between the BMA and the Government, and the BMA doctors withdrew their services from all public hospitals in Tasmania. Ratten was appointed Surgeon Superintendent at the Hobart General Hospital on 14th May 1917.

Ratten the Dentist

R ATTEN started his career as a dentist. He is said to have trained as a dental mechanic in Texas for three years but if you look at the timelines this does not seem possible; he is also said to have been apprenticed to a dentist in Sydney but there is no record of this.

On 19th December 1899 a newspaper article declared:

'Mr Victor R Ratten, eldest son of the Rev G W Ratten will leave Sydney in a few days and settle in Wyalong to commence the practice of his profession as a dentist'.

The next mention is on 19th January 1901 saying that he is making good progress from an injury.

'We are pleased to be able to state that Mr V R Ratten is making good progress towards recovery. The joint of his arm is now healed, but there is still trouble over the silver tubes. We sincerely hope that the latest difficulty will soon be overcome'.

On 1st February 1901 Ratten registered as a dentist in New South Wales under the new Dental Act of 1900, his only qualification for registration being that he was in practice before the passing of the Act.

This is no different to most new professions today when legislation is passed making it a requirement to be registered to legally practice. They are registered under a grandfathering clause. His registration was annotated 'c/o Mr S Hough, 59 Queen St. Brisbane', which seems to indicate that he was contemplating or had already made a move to Queensland.

On 25 June 1901 Ratten sold his practice in Wyalong NSW, the reason stated being ill health and his consequent inability to resume his professional duties. In September and November 1901 he was advertising his practice in Sydney. *'A Card. Mr V R Ratten. Surgeon Dentist. 'Beryldor', 139 Philip St. Sydney. Hours 9am till 5pm'.*

In October 1901 he advertised that he would be visiting Gympie in Queensland and would be available for consultations:

'Dr Ratten guarantees ABSOLUTELY PAINLESS Extractions and Fillings by the aid of the newly discovered Cataphoresis. Highest–class Dentistry, with all the latest improvements on moderate terms. CONSULTATIONS FREE. NIB. — The public of Gympie will have the opportunity of consulting a HIGHLY-qualified Dentist, who is thoroughly versed in all the latest methods of Painless Dentistry'.

So Ratten was advertising practices in Sydney and Gympie at the same time.

He then moved to Brisbane for reasons unknown, but possibly to be near his uncle Frederick William Ratten, who spent much of his married life in Queensland.

On 16th July 1903 he applied for registration as a dentist in Queensland, which required that applicants had attained the age of 21 years, were of good name and character and had engaged in the practice of dentistry in Queensland for two years prior to the proclamation of the Act. The Dental Board refused registration on the grounds that he did not satisfy the requirements and advised him that he could appeal to the Minister, as was his right.

'If the Board refuses to register any person as a dentist the Board shall if required by him state in writing the reasons for such refusal and such person may there upon appeal to the Minister and the Minister may after hearing such person and the Board dismiss the appeal or order the Board to register such person'.

The Board was obviously trying to be helpful because it approached the Crown Solicitor on 2nd October 1903 asking if provisional registration was possible; it was not.

Ratten appealed to the Minister, saying among other things that he was registered as a dentist in NSW, that he had practised as a dentist for seven years — five years in NSW and 22 months in Queensland — and that he had one of the largest practices in Brisbane with four assistants,

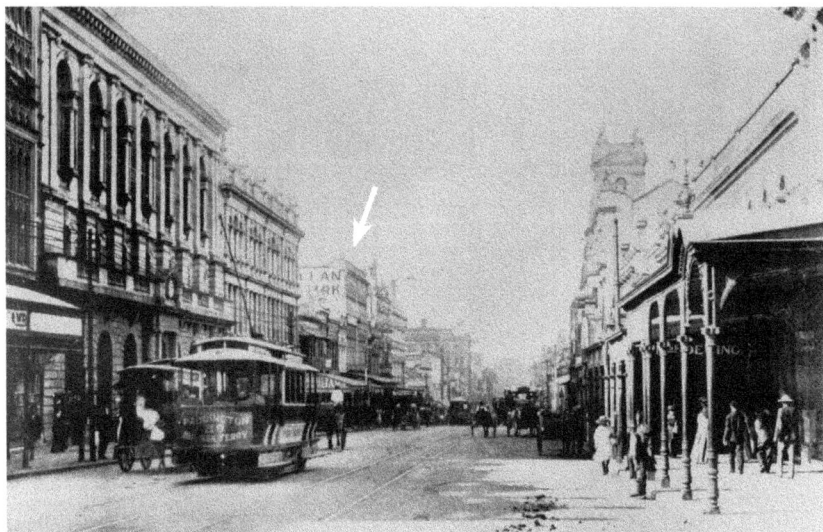

Ratten's Brisbane practice was housed in the building indicated by the arrow

and if he were not registered a considerable number of the public would suffer. Letters went back and forth between the Minister and the Dental Board.

The Board justified its decision, saying that registration in NSW was no qualification for registration in Queensland; that his 22 months' practice in Brisbane included seven months since the passing of the Dental Act; and that he had made statements in his advertisements which, in the opinion of the Board, were misleading and inaccurate. Ratten was becoming impatient.

On 14th November he wrote to the Minister, 'I would esteem it a personal favour if you would instruct the Dental Board to register me at an early date'.

Ratten said he wanted to go on holiday and leave his assistants in charge but that he could not unless he was registered. He told the Minister that he had carried out the Minister's wishes on advertising.

Ratten was registered as a dentist on 2nd December 1903. There was obviously a lot of activity behind the scenes and there are mentions of meetings between the Minister and Ratten. Practice addresses are given as 59, 128 and 156 Queen Street, Brisbane.

A promotional article appeared in the 21st December 1905 issue of the *Brisbane Courier*-headed 'The Ideal Dentists'.

'In October 1901 the Ideal Dentists commenced practice in Brisbane, bringing with them their new method of painless extraction. They first started in a suite of three rooms, but their practice increased to such an extent that they now have six rooms, including a large waiting room. Dr Ratten is the operating dental surgeon and is kept very busy. It is a great boon to have teeth extracted without pain or evil after effects and without the risk of an anaesthetic. Dr Ratten states that "The ideal Dentists" have to be very careful with the formula of the drugs they inject, in order to prevent anyone obtaining some of them in the hope of getting them analysed and so being able to use them. "The Ideal Dentists" carefully sterilise all their instruments. Every instrument, large or small, that is used on a patient is thoroughly boiled in water containing a little Lysol. By doing this the patient is secure from the risk of blood poisoning etc. With all their facilities for extracting teeth painlessly, the Ideal Dentists are great advocates of saving teeth where possible, and make a specialty of gold fillings, gold crowns, Davis crowns, and bridgework — i.e., teeth replaced without plates. In cases where a plate is necessary, however, they announce that they make it so light and thin by a new process that is hardly noticed by the wearer'.

Ratten, however, was not to remain for long as a dentist in Brisbane.

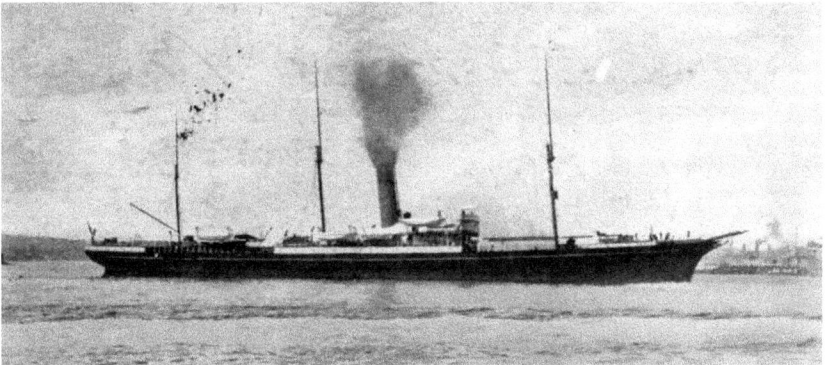

Quite suddenly and unexpectedly Ratten left Australia aboard the *Aorangi* on 3rd September 1906 for Vancouver. Advertisements for his practice continued, so the four assistants continued to run the practice — but for how long?

Upon his return to Australia in May 1907 Ratten soon commenced his new professional career as a doctor.

His name was removed from the dental register on 6th March 1917 for failure to pay the registration fee, which is around the time the dispute was arising in Hobart. He remained registered in NSW until 7th May 1928, his records annotated 'Address Unknown'.

American Medical Education

COLONIAL AMERICA had an apprenticeship medical education system and about 1860 they had developed several proprietary medical schools which were created to supplement the apprenticeship system.

This was exactly what happened in Tasmania in its early years. Medical students were apprenticed here and then went to one of the medical schools in the United Kingdom where they completed their training and received the medical qualification of that University or College if they passed. This applied until medical schools were established in Australia: University of Melbourne 1864; University of Sydney 1883; and University of Adelaide 1885.

In America entrance requirements were essentially nonexistent, other than the ability to pay the fees and if a qualification could not be earned, it was bought. Between 1870 and 1900 the number of medical schools more than doubled and in 1906 there were 162 schools operating.

American medical education at the turn of the 19th century was neither well organised nor well controlled and the American Medical Association did not have a list of medical schools at the time.

In 1910 the Carnegie Foundation reported on its extensive survey of medical education in the United States over five years:

'An enormous number of uneducated and ill trained medical practitioners, that there was a very large number of commercial schools, sustained in many cases by advertising methods through which a mass of unprepared youth was drawn into the study of medicine'.

In 1902 the American Medical Association decided to adopt an educational requirement for membership based on preliminary education and sufficient training, and established a permanent committee on medical education.

They rated colleges on the percentage of graduating students who failed the registering body's examinations. In the 1870s licensing boards had been established to certify medical schools and examine applicants for a licence to practise in that State. They were regarded as generally weak and ineffective and a few were viewed as corrupt. As late as 1906 thirteen states still granted medical licences to non-graduates.

There were five especially rotten spots, which included Illinois. In 1907 the Association reported on its review of 160 schools and found that 50 per cent were sufficiently equipped to teach modern medicine, 30 per cent were doing poor work and 20 per cent were unworthy of recognition. They further reported

'...found schools which are absolutely worthless, without any equipment for laboratory teaching, without any dispensaries, without any hospital facilities, some of which are no better equipped to teach medicine than is a Turkish bath establishment or barber shop'.

This was the environment when Ratten arrived in America.

Boston University established a homeopathic medical school in 1873, but homeopathy played a minor role in mainstream American medical education. Ratten's uncle, Arthur Ratten, obtained his medical qualification from the Boston University Medical School.

Harvey Medical College

RATTEN registered as a medical practitioner in South Australia and Tasmania based on a Diploma, Doctor of Medicine, from the Harvey Medical College, Chicago, dated 8th March 1907. There is no record of his having been a student there, nor was he a graduate — yet he had a student pass.

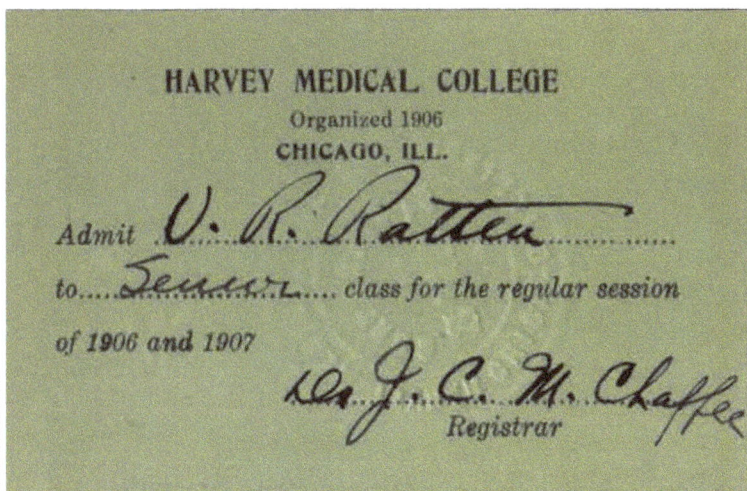

The Harvey Medical College had a somewhat chequered history; it was incorporated on 23rd November 1891, reincorporated on 14th August 1894, had its charter cancelled on 1st July 1902 and withdrawn on 5th March 1904.

In June 1905 the Harvey Medical College ceased active teaching, the building was demolished and it merged with the Jenner College. Ratten had not left Australia at this date. On 19th March 1907 the Harvey Medical College had its charter reinstated. It said that it expected to resume active business as a medical college, but it never did.

The issue is further confused by the incorporation in January 1907 of the Harvey Medical College and Hospital, which was housed in a rented office in the Fort Dearborn Bank building on the site of the old Harvey Medical College. This cannot be true because the bank building had opened in 1895. It had neither teaching nor laboratory facilities and was never recognised by the State of Illinois as entitling a graduate to practise in that state.

The Harvey Medical College and Hospital also had a chequered history; it was incorporated on 19th January 1907, changed its name to Jackson University on 2nd

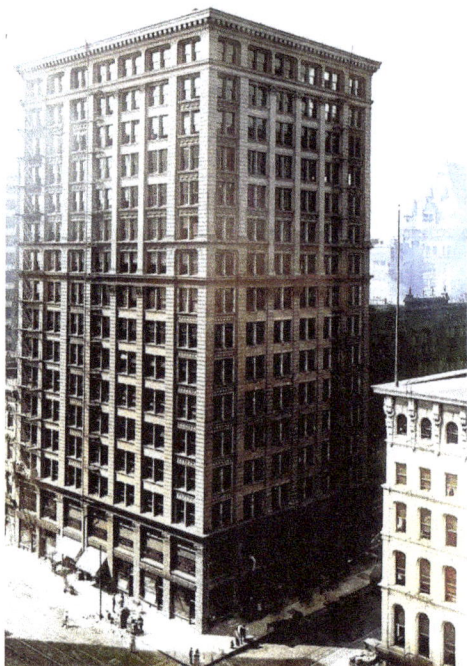

The Fort Dearborn building in Chicago

November 1908, changed it again to Jefferson University on 27th September 1909 and had its charter cancelled on 17th May 1912. Jackson and Jefferson Universities existed only as legally registered names.

Ratten could not have received a diploma from the Harvey Medical College on 8th March 1907 — his qualification was a fraud.

There were four signatories to his diploma, one being Dr William Gayle French, President of the Board of Directors, who had been convicted of selling bogus dental diplomas.

To practise legally a medical practitioner had to be registered in the State in which they intended to practice. Registration was granted by a government-appointed authority based on qualifications and training. The authority could even examine applicants if necessary.

Further suspicions as to the credibility of Ratten's qualification arose from the fact that Ratten did not register to practise in Illinois, where he had obtained his medical qualification, but in Texas. His certificate was dated 12th March 1907 and was illegal in that it was signed only by six of the nine members of the Board.

Until 12th July 1907 there were three separate licensing bodies in Texas, and Ratten was registered by the Homeopathic Board at its meeting on 4th-5th July 1907 when 415 people were registered. It was claimed that only eleven were given by examination, the rest having registered on credentials.

His certificate was signed on 12th March 1907, just days after the signing of his MD on 8th March 1907 and was not registered until a meeting of the Texas Board in July 1907, months after Ratten was back in Australia and registered here.

The Secretary of the Texas Board of Medical Examiners said in a letter dated 8th May 1920 that the majority of certificates were issued to very dubious applicants from every part of the United States. Many certificates were sold throughout Texas, Oklahoma, Arkansas and other states after they were outlawed. He also said that Ratten had written to him in 1920, asking for endorsement of his licence, which the Secretary refused.

So is this the true story? Dr French registered the Harvey Medical College and Hospital for $3000. It rented one room on the third floor of the Fort Dearborn Bank built on the site of the demolished Harvey Medical College. French realised that he could not provide a diploma MD from the Harvey Medical College and Hospital because it had only been in existence for two months, so he removed the words 'and Hospital' and provided a diploma MD from the Harvey Medical College which would have been legitimate — however, not since 1905, but that did not seem to worry him.

But what about the signatories to the diploma? We know about French. He was the instigator of the whole scam and was in trouble with the authorities for many years with selling false qualifications, immoral advertising, abortions and obtaining money under false pretences. He claimed to be the head of institutions that did not exist. A Dr H P Husley signed the diploma but no-one by that name could be traced and it was suggested it was a Dr Hurley, a physician of good standing, who maintained that he did not sign the certificate. The name Dr M A Brown also could not be traced If the diploma had been legitimate the names of the signatories would have been correct.

Sheffield

THE RURAL community of Sheffield, 29 kilometres from Devonport in the Kentish area, was settled in 1859. During World War I Sheffield had a population of 1076 and the Kentish agricultural region it serviced had 5112 inhabitants.

Ratten's time in Sheffield was seminal to his future career. It was here that he decided to become a surgeon, established a reputation as a successful one, and first found he could be accepted as important, socially and professionally successful.

His first practice was on the corner of Main and Henry Streets behind the current Murial's corner craft shop and next to the Chinese restaurant.

He also rented a house off Main Street, where the visitor centre now stands, to open a hospital.

In 1909 he bought the block diagonally opposite his practice and built an eleven-roomed house which the locals said would add beauty to the place. The house faced Main Street and the adjoining surgery faced Henry Street.

It was said to be built on the most sanitary principles and fitted with every modern convenience, although later there were complaints about its drains.

He also built an entertainment room separate from the house which had an open fire and two large billiard tables. There was a concrete swimming pool and when the telephone was connected it made local news.

In 1910, soon after his arrival, Ratten put a public notice in the local newspaper:

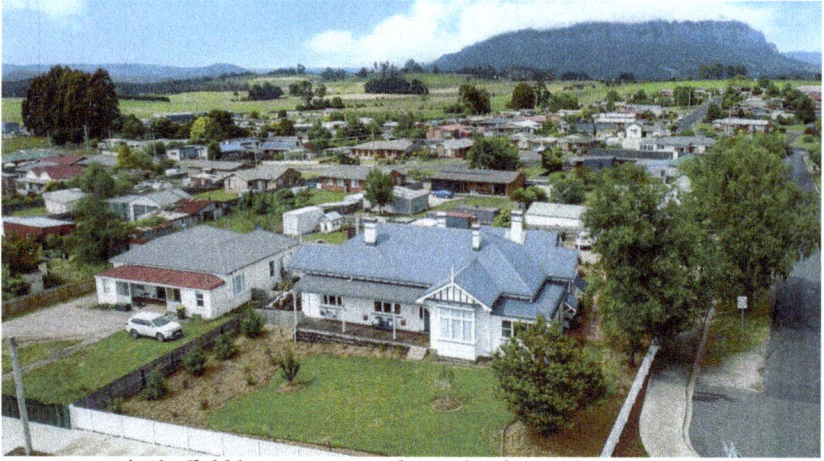

Ratten's Sheffield house as it is today — his former hospital on the left

'*Dr Ratten desires to contradict that [it] is being persistently circulated in Sheffield that his practice is for sale and that he is leaving Sheffield. Such a thing is furthermost from his mind, and he has no intention of leaving the district*'.

This might have been genuine — or perhaps it was merely a promotional stunt.

In 1912 he had approval to build a nine-room hospital next to his house, but this did not meet with universal acceptance and local opinion

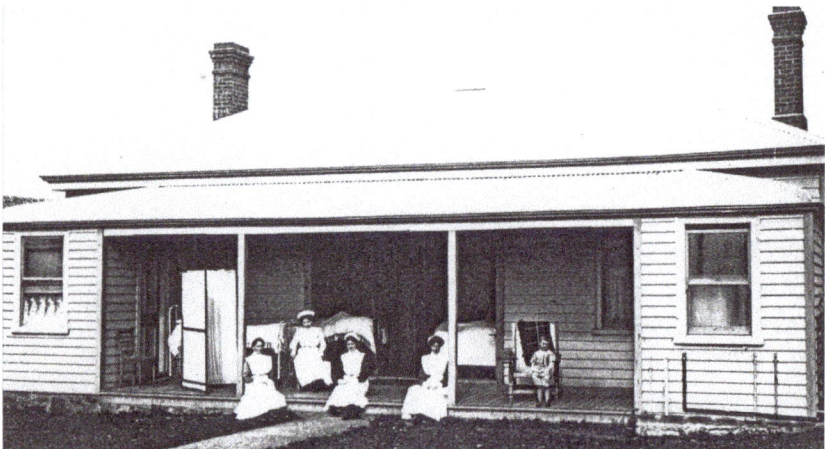

Ratten's Sheffield hospital

was that it should be further from the heart of town. It was said that it was expected that the doctor's venture would be a remunerative one.

Dyer, a local historian, described Ratten as a very talented extrovert who seemed to end up at the centre of Kentish life.

'Having just lived and trained in the affluent and progressive country of the USA this energetic and confident young doctor introduced a new style of medical practice to this sleepy country town that jolted this rural community into the 20th century'.

Soon after his arrival there was a meeting to support the establishment of an Australian-trained nurses' association in Tasmania to set standards for training; it was stressed that it needed the cooperation of doctors if it was to succeed. A proposed grandfather clause stipulated that nurses would be eligible for registration if they could get positive references from three doctors.

The range and type of work that came Ratten's way was probably much the same as a rural general practitioner sees today, but the difference would be that Ratten had to cope alone — he couldn't send a patient to the nearest major hospital by ambulance, nor did he have today's facilities and equipment.

In those days before antibiotics infections were a problem; patients with infectious diseases such as diphtheria were transferred to the Devon Hospital in Latrobe as Ratten refused to keep such patients in his hospital.

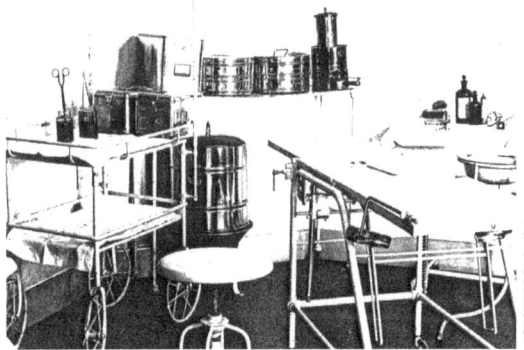

Ratten's Sheffield surgery

There were many cases of injuries — lacerations, fractures sometimes resulting in death — and Ratten dealt with all of these. Either the patient was brought to him or he went to the patient by car; and if there was no road or the road was impassable, on horseback.

Sporting injuries such as horse racing falls and gun accidents were frequent, along with snakebites, drownings, falling trees, chopping accidents, splinters with infections and suicides brought about by failed harvests.

Much more rarely encountered today are the injuries typical of that horse-drawn age — horse kicks, falls from a broken stirrup, traps colliding, running away or capsizing, cart and trap shafts breaking, horses and bullock teams bolting, burns from carbide lamps and even a bursting yeast bottle.

Pneumonias, seizures, dropsies and rheumatic fevers were much less treatable and patients with serious internal maladies had to be sent to Launceston. This was all fertile experience for Ratten, and he capitalised on it.

Ratten loved using his surgical skills and nearly any excuse was good enough for an operation. Appendicitis was the fashionable disease and the epidemic of appendicitis cases which coincided with his early years in Sheffield was probably due to Ratten's enthusiasm for the knife. It was openly said by some of the locals that some of the appendicectomies were probably unnecessary — but who argues with a doctor?

Ratten had to get surgical experience somewhere and one of the local stories was that there wasn't a rabbit left in Sheffield with an appendix.

Only one fatality was recorded. At no time is there mention of who gave the anaesthetic — probably Ratten himself.

Ratten was not admired by everyone, and once someone hung a sign on his door: 'Butcher Ratten'.

He also had a public health role, advising on safety issues with the Mount Roland Hall and concerns about water supply from the town creek.

Social issues included dealing with the consequences of infant death, securing pensions for eligible people, such as a Crimean War veteran, and publicity about the oldest resident in the state about who — notwithstanding all theories to the contrary — had been a heavy drinker and smoker for many years.

He also had a role as an expert witness in court, appearing in cases such as an offence against a girl in consequence of which she was 'in a certain condition'; failure to support an illegitimate child; assault by biting off part of an ear; and the theft of rabbit traps.

Ratten hosted dignitaries, such as the American Ambassador when he visited Sheffield, and was a medical officer in the 12th Australian Light Horse and the 23rd Army Corps, where he held the rank of Captain.

He joined the Horticultural Society, the Ploughing Association and the Rifle Club and a was member of the local Masonic Lodge.

Ratten distinguished himself in sports — he was in the cricket team, which held such events as married versus singles and smokers versus non-smokers — and a record still stands: 99 rabbits trapped during a game. He was prominent in tennis and fishing clubs and set up a local football competition, the Wilmot Football Association, donating a perpetual V R Ratten shield, and challenged the best in the area in billiards and pigeon shooting.

Ratten was one of the few car owners in the area. Roads in those times were narrow, steep and rough with many unbridged stream crossings passable in flood times only with difficulty. He had one of his cars modified to carry an improvised stretcher.

With the outbreak of World War I he was commissioned as a temporary Captain (Medical Officer) in the 12th battalion, Australian Imperial Forces on 20th August 1914. On 20th October 1914 he sailed on the SS *Geelong,* the first ship to carry troops as part of the expeditionary force. His family remained in Sheffield with Dr David Hamilton as locum for the practice. He embarked in Egypt to return to Australia on 5th February 1915, acting on board as medical officer to troops being invalided back to Australia on the hired transport *Kyarra.* He disembarked to the Third Military District in Melbourne on 11th March 1915.

He must have been restless and soon after decided to move to Hobart. On 2nd April 1916 at a farewell attended by 40 people at the Caledonian Hotel he was presented with a wall clock and a case of pipes.

Father Patrick Hayes, the Irish catholic priest for 56 years from St Mary's Presbytery in Burnie, was unable to attend but in his apology expressed his appreciation of the qualities of the genial doctor whose reputation as a medical man and surgeon had spread through northern Tasmania, adding that his sporting and social qualities were an asset for any town; he was full of praise for Ratten — except for Ratten's sotto voce remarks when things went awry on the tennis court.

Ratten retained an interest in Sheffield for some years. He sold his vacant hospital in 1917 to Dr Herbert Tredennick, a dentist from Melbourne, who occupied it for the next 40 years and his home in 1920 to Dr Henry Jackson who lived there until 1927. The next owner was Dr William Firth, who named the house 'Coldale' and remained there until 1946. The current owners have renamed it 'Ratten House'. When Ratten sold his house he bought the oldest building in Sheffield, Padman's Hall opposite the Methodist Church, housed his two billiards tables there and made it into a billiard saloon. It closed in about 1929.

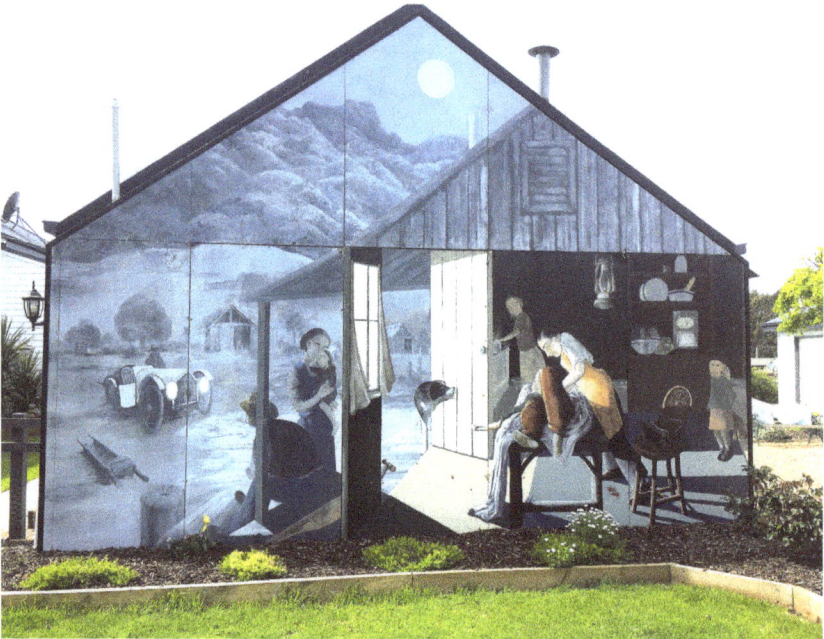

Sheffield is noted for its many murals, which bring many visitors to the town and this one on the front of what was once Ratten's private billiard saloon, depicts him attending the victim of a logging accident. He has positioned his car to use the headlights to illuminate his task. The calendar in the mural tells us it is in 1910, the year in which the main dwelling was completed.
Dr Ratten practised in this house until the outbreak of World War I 'when his services as a surgeon were required overseas'.

Ratten's Military Career

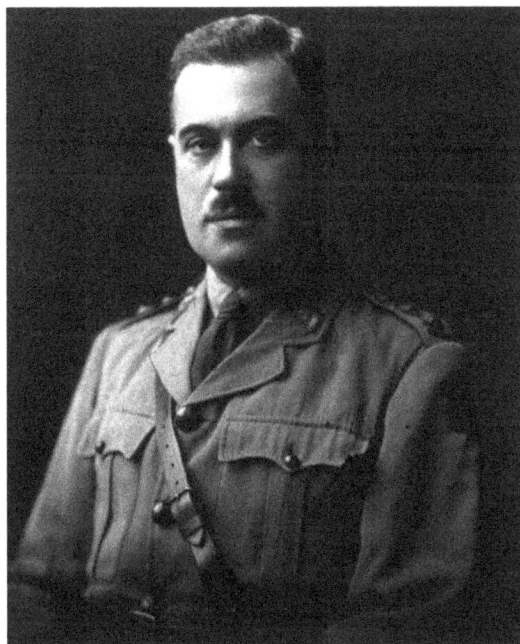

AUTHOR'S COLLECTION

R ATTEN'S involvement with the Army may have started at his father's school in Port Fairy, where the cadets were a feature of the College — '...with uniforms, Franchi rifles, drums and bugles. The cadets had a fine time; trips to various towns, Hamilton, Portland etc and engaging in shooting and other competitions. *(The Age* 30th May 1936)

Compulsory naval or military training was introduced for all men between the ages of 12 and 60 in 1911. Those between 12 and 18 joined the cadets and those over 18 had to join the Citizen Military Forces, which included some volunteers. Men could not be forced to serve overseas. This scheme was abolished in 1929.

In 1909 Ratten was a captain in the Australian Army Medical Corps and served as medical officer to the 12th Australian Light Horse. In 1912 he was appointed to attend the 26th Light Horse and the 23rd Army Medical Corps encamped in the district.

The *Examiner* newspaper reported on 18th April 1914 that Ratten had offered his services to the Empire and on 28th August that 'the band paraded in front of the doctor's residence and played patriotic airs'.

He applied for a commission on 25th August and was appointed to the 12th Battalion 4th Infantry Brigade as regimental medical officer.

Ratten urgently needed a locum and fortunately there was a single graduate from Glasgow, Dr David Hamilton, who had recently been in New Norfolk and was available,. He reopened St Helen's Hospital and remained in Sheffield after Ratten returned, finally leaving in 1918.

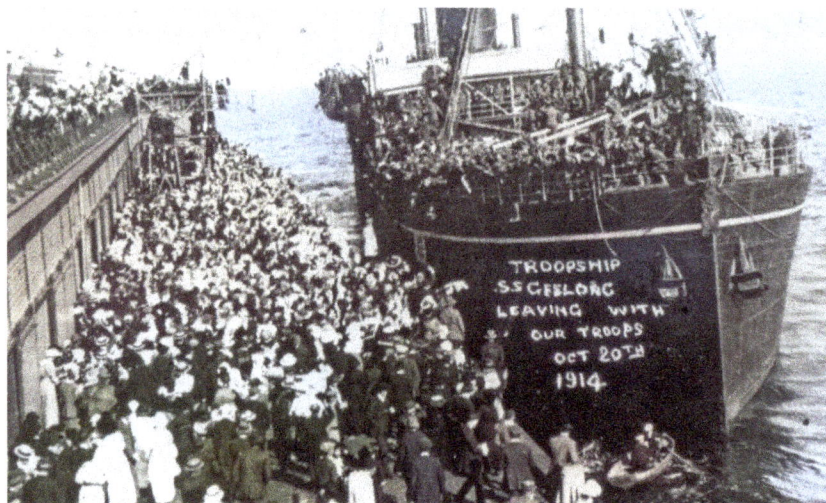

TROOPSHIP SS GEELONG LEAVING WITH OUR TROOPS OCT 20TH 1914.

Things moved quickly and Captain Ratten was in the first contingent of the World War I, embarking on the transport SS *Geelong* on 20th October 1914. The *Geelong* arrived in Albany on 26 October and left in a convoy of 36 transport vessels and two cruisers, which stretched seven and a half miles. They arrived in Cairo on 10th December 1914 via Colombo, Aden, Port Said and Alexandria. They began company training on 14th December and battalion training on 1st February 1915.

On 5th December 1914 the hospital ship *Kyarra* left Melbourne for Egypt; one of the doctors on board was Major John Mitchell Young Stewart and he was expected to return with the *Kyarra* to Australia.

When the *Kyarra* departed from Egypt on 5th February 1915 to return to Australia it carried several hundred servicemen, including

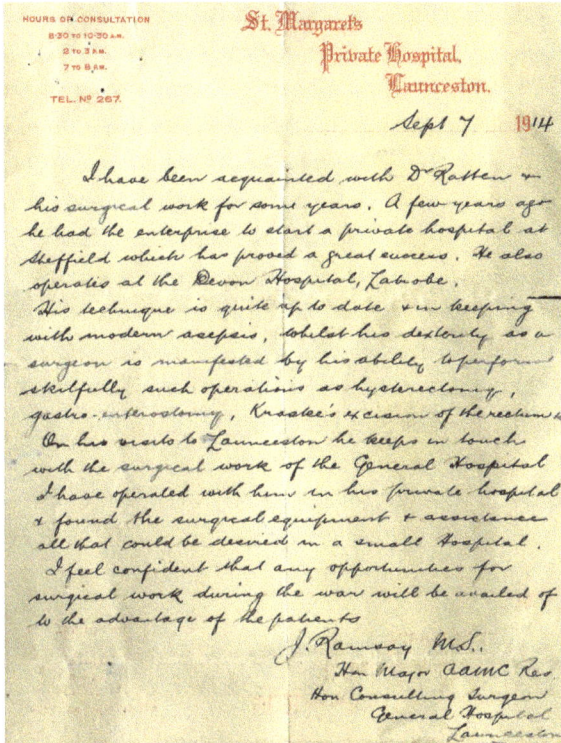

A reference provided to support Ratten's enlistment,
transcribed below

St. Margaret's Private Hospital, Launceston
Sept 7 1914

'I have been acquainted with Dr Ratten and his surgical work for some years. A few years ago he had the enterprise to start a private hospital at Sheffield which has proved a great success. He also operates at the Devon Hospital, Latrobe.

'His technique is quite up to date and in keeping with modern asepsis, whilst his dexterity as a surgeon is manifested by his ability to perform skilfully such operations as hysterectomy, gastroenterostomy, Knacke's excision of the rectum etc.

'On his visits to Launceston he keeps in touch with the surgical work of the General Hospital.

'I have operated with him in his private hospital and found the surgical equipment and assistance all that could be desired in a small hospital.

'I feel confident that any opportunities for surgical work during the war will be availed of to the advantage of the patients.'

J. Ramsay MS
Hon. Major AAMC Res
Hon Consulting Surgeon
General Hospital
Launceston

those ill or injured during training or being returned for serious breaches of discipline, one doctor and nine nurses. Ratten replaced Major Stewart on *Kyarra's* return passage with Major Stewart staying in Egypt, taking part in the Gallipoli landing and serving for the duration of the war.

An Australian sergeant made a significant remark: 'At present there are 70,000 troops camped in and around Cairo so you can just imagine what things are like, the hospitals are full, and you can take it from me that for every 100 men who are invalided from here (either to Australia or elsewhere) there are 99 who are victims of their own folly and the filthy state of the women'.

Dr Nigel Abbott told me that Ratten was invalided back to Australia with a social disease, not just escorting patients back as stated. When I was researching Ratten's Army career the Army refused to release his personal files, even though there were no living next of kin at the time.

On 11th March 1915 the *Kyarra* arrived back in Melbourne and on 13th March Ratten's appointment was terminated.

On 19th March the *North Western Advocate and Emu Bay Times* reported:

'*Captain Dr Ratten, of Sheffield, medical officer in charge of the Australian soldiers invalided home by the hospital ship* Kyarra *arrived from Melbourne by the* Loongana *today. Captain Ratten said that all the men who returned to Tasmania were sent back owing to illness and not for breaches of discipline. The Australians had created a very favourable impression in Egypt and the conduct of the Tasmanians had been excellent. They had also paid great attention to their training and were now soldiers. The men were very anxious to get to the front and he was sure they would render a good account of themselves. Dr Ratten is under orders to proceed to the front and will leave Melbourne shortly with a body of troops, probably reinforcements for the previous contingents.*'

A further report in the *North Western Advocate* on 20th March 1915 said:

'*Dr V R Ratten who went to Egypt with the First Australian Expeditionary Force, returned to Melbourne this week aboard the hospital ship* Kyarra, *and is now spending a few days on furlough at his home in Sheffield, prior to again returning to take up his position with the Australian RAMC'.*

These two reports indicate that it was expected that Ratten would be returning to the front when this could not be the case because his appointment had been terminated.

Ratten appeared before an Army medical board on 22nd May 1915, and it related to injuries he sustained in January and April 1915 to his left shoulder.

'He has old disability of left arm due to resection of the head of the humerus 18 years following an accident in Wyalong in 1901 in consequence of which there is loss of action of the deltoid muscle.

'He said that his horse stumbled in Mena and he fell on his affected shoulder. The effects from this have practically recovered.

'On his return to Sheffield he was cranking a car which backfired in consequence of which there was swelling, bruising and pain in the scar of the old operation and some loss of function. The swelling and bruising have disappeared but there remains he said some loss of function of central fibres of deltoid muscle. Now abduction of the arm beyond 45 degrees is impossible.'

The Board reported that beyond his own statements there was no evidence of his having suffered any recent injury. 'All the disability is due in our opinion to the injury 18 years ago'. It said that he was only incapacitated by the results of that injury.

How was it, then, that he passed the medical examination to get into the army? And how was it that he was an accomplished sportsman, particularly in tennis, all his life? His medical certificate made no mention of his injury 18 years previously and stated that he was capable of bearing the fatigue incident to military service.

He was awarded the 1914-15 Star, the British War Medal and the Victory Medal and was placed on the list of retired officers with the rank of major.

Ratten's left arm was a recurring problem. He was involved in a car accident in 1933 and hurt his left arm; Dr Gaha is reported to have operated to save it.

During World War II he was involved with army medical boards until

1941, was a surgeon at the 111th Australian General Hospital, Hobart from December 1941 and performed camp duties until 1945. He remained a member of the Returned Sailors and Soldiers imperial League of Australia (RSSILA), now the RSL, all his life.

Resolution of the Dispute
1920-1930

THE DISPUTE, which involved all public hospitals in Tasmania was resolved for the Launceston General Hospital in 1924. The surgeon superintendent there was Dr Ireland, who was considered easy to get on with. They didn't have Ratten.

From 1917 to 1930 the Hobart General Hospital was staffed by Ratten, Dr MacGowan, Dr Crowther and a series of medical officers which at various stages included Dr W G C Clark, the two Gaha brothers, Dr Tom Gaha and Dr John Francis (Frank, Stymie) Gaha, and Dr B M Carruthers.

The Hobart General Hospital expanded over the years and there does not appear to have been much concern about the service it provided.

It appears that Matron Gluyas (pictured right) gave most of the anaesthetics for Ratten's surgery and was by all accounts quite competent. But all was not as it seemed and one recommendation following a hospital inquiry was that there should always be a second medical practitioner in the operating theatre in addition to Ratten during surgery. She resigned in 1931 soon after the BMA returned to the hospital.

But there were personality clashes and complaints about

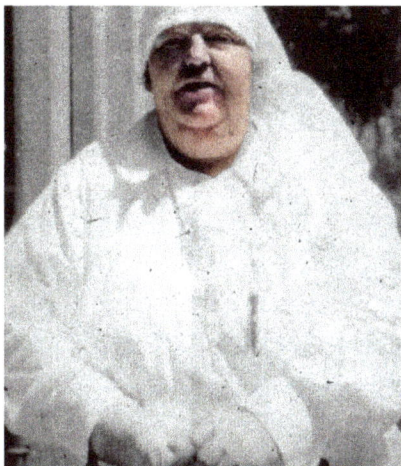

administration. Ratten would be frequently quoted favourably in the newspapers, praising his care of patients; BMA doctors would challenge and criticise Ratten's management of patients at every opportunity. There was a well-publicised investigation of the health of a patient by the name of Petterd, which led to outside medical practitioners appearing before the Board.

At this time Ratten did not have the right of private practice and there were complaints about him receiving fees for consultations and about missing radium which could have been used by Ratten in the treatment of his patients. Dr Clark, a resident medical officer with an American medical qualification, was suspended for insubordination, having accused Ratten of carrying on an illicit practice .

Dr Clark took the Government to court on the grounds of unfair dismissal and won, receiving a healthy payment of £675.

The BMA continued to fight to return to the Hospital, bitterly regretting the lost years and seeing itself as being in the wilderness. As Dr Clifford Craig remarked, the General Hospital was the spiritual home of medicine and nothing else could replace it .

In addition to continued efforts by the BMA to get back their appointments at the Hospital, the medical profession attempted to increase private hospital beds so that they could continue to treat their private patients.

By this stage the BMA would have been glad to settle the dispute. It had learnt two lessons: resignation is dangerous in that you lose any voice you have; and it is impossible to fight a government which can make and change laws.

It took many years of negotiation before the dispute was over and BMA doctors returned to the Hospital. Those considered responsible for this were Dr Frank Fay MC, who had a wise and moderate attitude, for the BMA, and Dr Stymie Gaha and Dr Carruthers for the Government.

Dr Gaha was to go on to become the first ever Minister for Health in the Ogilvie Labor Government. Dr Carruthers became the first Director of Public Health.

There were many meetings at Hospital Board level but invariably the Government had to be consulted before any decision could be made.

Dr Fay pointed out how backward the Hospital was in a report to the Hospital Board which was published in full in the *Mercury* on 15th June 1928. He compared the staff at the Melbourne Hospital with staff at the Hobart General hospital. He chose the Melbourne Hospital as an example of a public hospital with honorary staff. It had 460 beds, just double those at the Hobart General Hospital, and 104 medical staff compared to the Hobart General Hospital with five. He went on to say that all the specialties were included in the departments of medicine and surgery at the Melbourne Hospital. To support his argument about specialisation he quoted Dr Hogg, the recently retired President of the BMA: 'Long past is the day when at a hospital a medical man was a general physician and surgeon treating all and every form of disease.'

Dr Fay argued that the advantage to the Hospital would be better treatment and facilities, specialised medical care, good resident training and lower costs. The Hospital could be a clinical school for medical undergraduates and might encourage the holding of medical congresses in Tasmania. Additionally, patients would have choice, something that was denied them. He believed that medical practitioners in Hobart could supply honorary staff in all specialties — surgery, medicine, ophthalmology, ear nose and throat surgery, gynaecology, anaesthesia, radiology, venereology and pathology.

Finally, Dr Fay pointed out that with staffing similar to the Launceston General Hospital — that is, a surgeon superintendent and six to eight full-time resident medical officers — total salaries would be considerably less than those then paid at the Hobart General Hospital.

Following Dr Fay's oral report to the Board, Ratten was asked about the adequacy of the Hospital staff. The minutes record: 'In reply to a question asked the surgeon superintendent stated that in his opinion the Hospital was fully staffed both as regards medical and nursing requirements'. Ratten felt that comparison with the Broken Hill Hospital was a better comparison than the Melbourne Hospital.

The Board supported Dr Fay and following many meetings the hurdles were overcome, and the BMA agreed to return to the Hospital on 22nd May 1930, against Ratten's wishes.

Private Hospitals in Hobart

AFTER the dispute in 1917 began, the BMA became increasingly aware of its dependence on the Hobart General Hospital for experience and for continued professional development. St Johns Hospital was a homeopathic hospital and therefore not really available for mainstream doctors, and St Helen's Hospital was probably regarded as Ratten's. Apart from these there were several small nursing homes and hospitals but nothing of significance. To overcome this deficit and not guessing how long the dispute would last, the BMA approached the Catholic Church.

On 28th December 1923 Dr E Brettingham Moore wrote to the Little Company of Mary asking about the possibility of their establishing a hospital in Hobart. This did not eventuate until 1941, when Calvary Hospital admitted its first patients. There was at this time the Hobart Homeopathic Hospital, which is now the St John s campus of Calvary Hospital and St Helens Hospital.

The Hobart Homeopathic Hospital was opened in 1899 and, interestingly, the rise of homeopathy in Hobart was one of the reasons for the establishment of the medical section of the Royal Society of Tasmania. It is recorded in the minutes of its meeting of 23rd March 1898:

'It was resolved that the Society is of the opinion that no legally qualified medical practitioner is justified in meeting professionally a homeopathic or any other irregular practitioner.'

In 1930 the Hospital faced mounting financial difficulties and was taken over by the St Johns Hospital Association, which was associated with the Anglican Church. In 1935 a new wing was established and in 1940 additional buildings were added so that in 1941 the Hospital had 64 beds.

St Helen's Hospital at 186 Macquarie Street was first recorded as a hospital there in 1919 when Constance Rout and Jeannie Campbell were listed as the owner-occupiers. Originally it was the site of the Royal Oak inn.

The original house was built in 1886 for Dr Edward Giblin by Henry Hunter, the renowned architect who was responsible for many of Hobart's fine buildings. Dr Giblin consulted from these rooms.

The building was sold to Dr John Edgar Wolfhagen in 1898, and it was his private residence until he sold it to Ratten in 1916, who consulted there. St Helens was a general and obstetric hospital of some 12 beds and was registered as a training school for nurses. After the death of Miss Campbell in 1931 and the retirement of Miss Rout in 1936 Ratten repurchased the property. The history and the transactions raise the question: did Ratten finance Misses Campbell and Rout in their purchase of St Helens in 1919, or did Ratten own the hospital all this time? It was also most opportune that Miss Rout

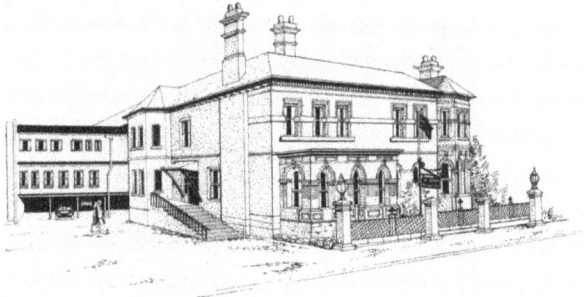

retired in 1936 — it coincided with Ratten's resignation as surgeon superintendent at the Hobart General Hospital. Matron Stafford was at St Helens from 1948 to 1951 and Matron Milner from 1951 to 1955. There was concern about the viability of the Hospital and it closed for a time.

The Government became actively involved in discussions with interested parties and in 1957 it bought St Helens from Ratten and undertook repairs and renovations. It was then bought by Dr Matysek in 1968, by Australian Hospital Care in1983 and eventually by Healthscope, who provided mental health beds and a mother and baby unit. It closed in June 2023 when maintenance of the ageing building became unsustainable. The government of the day ruled out buying the hospital.

One remaining mystery is why Ratten named both his hospitals in Sheffield and Hobart St Helens.

Resolution of the Dispute
1930-1936

A FTER the return of the BMA doctors to the hospital the dispute about the administration of the hospital continued unabated, as did disagreements between Ratten and the staff, but there was an improvement in the range of services the hospital provided.

Some of these changes were due to the influence of the BMA and the increase in medical practitioners in the hospital but there were other factors, such as increased scrutiny of everything that went on in the hospital, which included how Ratten was performing as surgeon superintendent as well as instability at board level — there were four different chairmen between 1930 and 1936.

A progressive government appointed the first Minister of Health, Dr Stymie Gaha, and the first Director of Public Health, Dr Carruthers. A deputy Superintendent was appointed and a new hospital was planned. New X-ray equipment and the appointment of a pathologist improved diagnostic services and the hospital gained a dietician, an almoner (social worker) and a crippled children's clinic. Medical colleges were being established and they changed attitudes to standards, teaching, training and specialist qualifications.

Dr Stymie Gaha (1894-1966) was a great supporter of Ratten since the early 1920s, when he was appointed a medical officer (honorary) at the hospital. When the BMA agreed to return to the hospital Gaha was required to apply for one of the new honorary positions; he refused, saying that he had originally been appointed for life but was unable to provide supporting documentation. He must have been appointed to one of the positions because he is recorded as retiring at the compulsory age of 60 on 22nd December 1953.

There were two Royal Commissions into the administration of the Hospital in 1931 and 1935 and in 1933 a special inquiry by the Board. The Hospital secretary was suspended for withholding matters of importance from the board chairman. The Auditor-General reported adversely on the hospital and several officers were dismissed. Radium had gone missing again. Board discussions about Ratten's contract showed some divisions. When Premier Ogilvie overruled the Board's attempt to engage Ratten as a part-time surgeon, the majority of the Board resigned, including Dr Fay who had done so much to resolve the dispute. In his resignation letter, which he refused to withdraw, he talked of the 'dictatorial action of the Premier which denies the board of any semblance of administrative power and in effect means that for the future becomes merely a convenient instrument for registering the wishes of the premier however detrimental they may be to the welfare of the hospital'.

Ratten refused to support the appointment of Matron Lade, the superintendent of nursing, and he charged her with wilfully disobeying a lawful command of himself as the surgeon superintendent. After a lot of conflict, including public meetings, she was dismissed.

Inevitably, relationships between Ratten and the honorary staff were strained, with concern expressed about access to the operating theatre for honoraries. Father O'Donnell, the chairman of the board from 1935 to 1936, was one of Ratten's fiercest opponents.

The board became increasingly suspicious of Ratten and questioned him about missing reports and how Mr Ogilvie, when Leader of the Opposition, had obtained copies of letters and quoted from them in the House of Assembly. Ratten was reminded of his responsibility to assist residents to gain experience and that he was required to be present on Board meeting days. He was told that he should comment on reports only to the Board and not to the public.

Ratten was again in trouble for his habit of ordering surgical instruments and equipment before seeking approval. He was in further trouble for supplying coal to the hospital from Catamaran Coal, a company of which he was a director and majority shareholder. This deal, which was contrary to the Hospitals Act, was negotiated with the hospital secretary without the board's approval or knowledge; the board was prepared to prosecute him. The Auditor-General saw this as merely a technical offence, but the Solicitor-General viewed it as a matter of considerable magnitude and grave importance. Ratten's pay was suspended but he was allowed to continue operating. The suspension was later rescinded.

Premier Ogilvie, who was overseas at this time, said in a letter to Ratten; 'Many thanks for your chatty letter. I feel quite sure that the hospital business will come all right in the end'.

Matters came to a head when the Board accused Ratten of 'neglect of duty and other things' and asked for his response. The Board launched an inquiry which had many meetings and heard much evidence, but before it finished Ratten intimated that he was prepared to terminate his contract and take a part-time appointment on certain conditions.

On 10th June 1936 the Premier discussed the situation with the Board and said that as he had already removed two boards he would sooner let Ratten go than to have to remove a third.

On 26th June the hospital held a farewell ceremony for Ratten and three nurses. He was presented with a combined book and instrument case. Of the three nurses, two were leaving to work at St Helens Hospital — one as a sister and the other as matron.

The minutes of the meeting in June 1936 recorded:

'As Dr Victor Richard Ratten has at his own request relinquished the position of Surgeon Superintendent of this hospital in order to take a position of part-time surgeon with the right of private practice the Board orders that a minute be placed on its records in recognition of the valued services rendered to this hospital by Dr Victor Richard Ratten as Surgeon Superintendent during the past 19 years'.

Ratten was then aged 58 and his departure was regarded as more of a gain than a loss. Premier Ogilvie, who had just returned from an overseas trip with Stymie Gaha, decided to replace the Board with a commission of three chaired by Dr Carruthers, the Director of Public Health. O'Donnell, who was increasingly in conflict with Ogilvie, firmly resisted this move, so Ogilvie changed the number to five members and reverted to calling it a Board. The new Board took office on 1st December 1936.

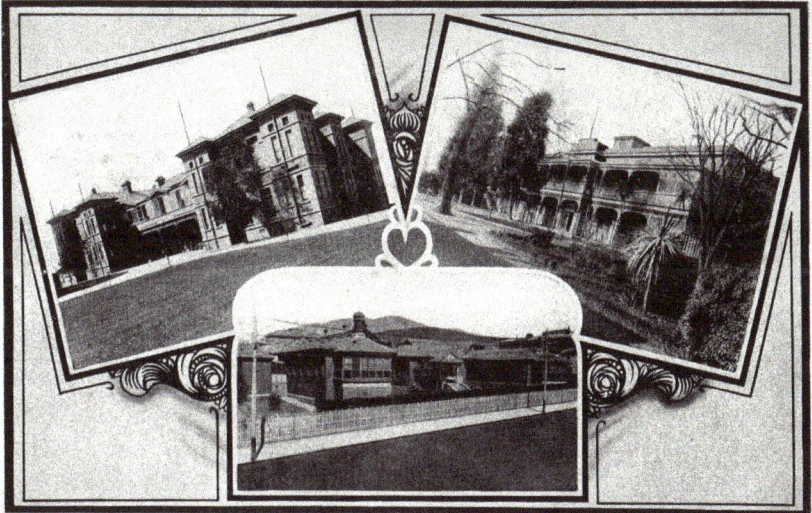

Certificates awarded to nurses in the 1930s included these images of the Hobart Public Hospital prior to the conferral of 'Royal' in its name.

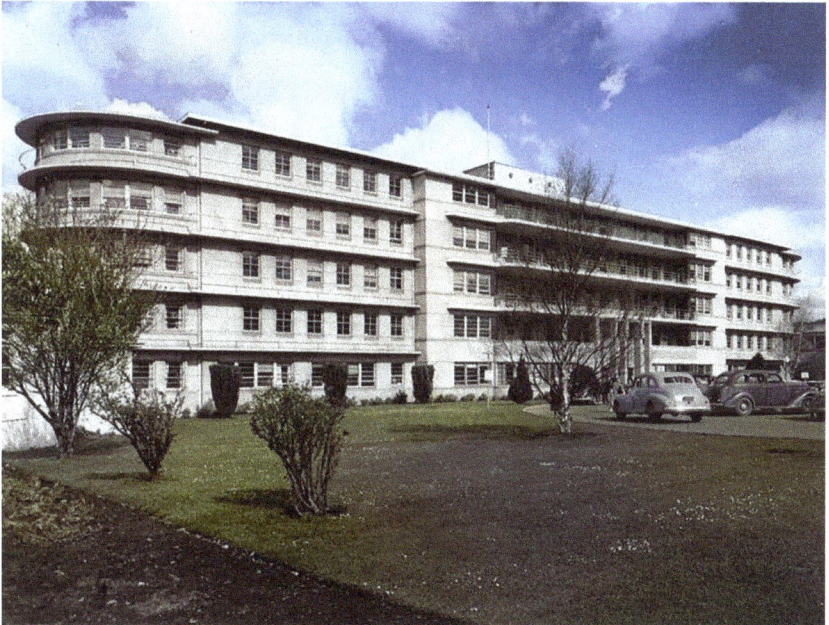

The new Royal Hobart Hospital shortly after Ratten's resignation in 1936

Father O'Donnell

FATHER Thomas Joseph (Tommy) O'Donnell, who was born in Victoria on 3rd August 1876 and died in Hobart on 3rd September 1949, was a passionate man.

Tasmanians saw him as one who stood for the underdog and who also believed that there were two sides to every question — his and the wrong one.

O'Donnell was chairman of the Hospital Board from 1935 to 1936 when Ratten resigned, and he had known Ratten and his family in the past.

In 1907 he was curate in Latrobe and a board member of the Devon Hospital not far from Ratten in Sheffield. In 1909 he was in Stanley where Ratten's father was a curate in the Anglican church. In 1921 he was involved in the Chrissie Venn murder trial along with Ratten and Ogilvie.

His life was more than spectacular. He was ordained after studying in Dublin and back in Australia he went on an interstate speaking tour supporting conscription.

In 1915 he was in Stanley and was friendly with the family of Joe Lyons, then a member of the Tasmanian House of Assembly. Lyons, a Catholic, became engaged to Methodist Enid Burnell from Burnie. Father O'Donnell assisted Enid's conversion to Catholicism and agreed to marry them in Wynyard, part of the Stanley parish. Enid resided in the Burnie parish which was the responsibility of Father Hayes. Father O'Donnell and Father Hayes were not the closest of friends and a disagreement arose with Father Hayes claiming the right to conduct the marriage.

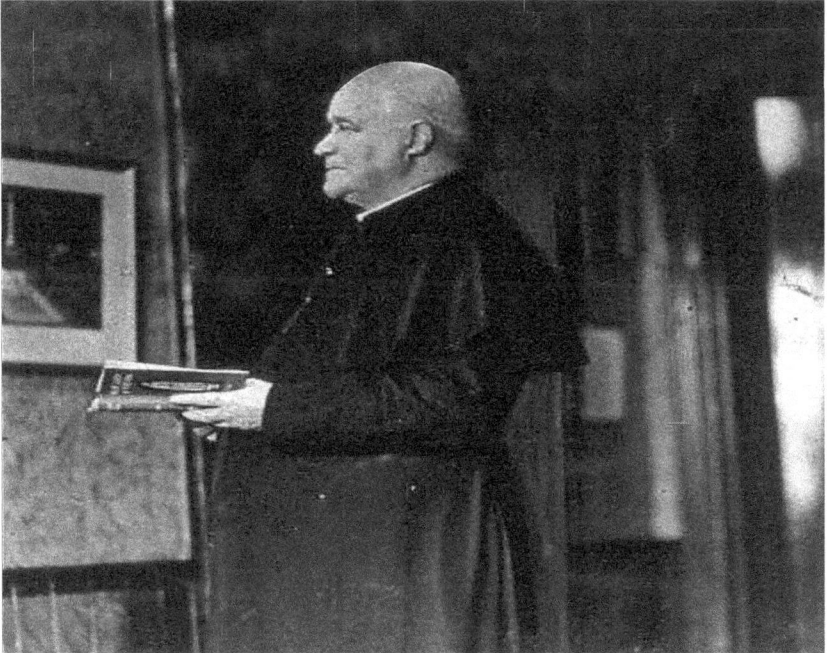

Under canon law it was the responsibility of Father Hayes. Father O'Donnell's response: 'I'm going to marry you and what's more, when I've married you the Pope himself can't unmarry you.' He married them.

There were consequences. It was argued out in Rome in the ecclesiastical courts of the Church and led to a revision of canon law covering marriage throughout the Catholic world.

He joined the AIF as chaplain with the rank of captain on 22nd February 1918 and on 14th October 1919 he was arrested in Ireland for traitorous and disloyal language about the King and British policy in Ireland, removed to Britain, incarcerated in the Tower of London, tried in the Guildhall by a general court martial on 26th-27th November and acquitted, though not honourably.

His stated aim had been to hand over to Sinn Feinners a pistol presented to supporters of the Irish rebel John Mitchell in Van Diemen's Land.

Australian Prime Minister W M 'Billy' Hughes cabled protests to the British Government and messages of support to O'Donnell. His case was raised in the House of Commons.

Returning to Tasmania, he continued in the ministry, was a known supporter of sport, and was a board member of several public hospitals.

He refused to attend the opening of the new Royal Hobart Hospital when he learned that his name had been removed from the foundation stone.

Stymie Gaha, questioned about O'Donnell, replied 'Will no one rid me of this turbulent priest?' — a phrase attributed to Henry II of England.

O'Donnell had been a supporter of Ogilvie and the Labor government but turned against them and in 1937, prior to an election, sent a letter to electors condemning the government and particularly Gaha.

The Qualities of a Surgeon

WHAT is a good surgeon? What makes a good surgeon? Much has been written in medical journals and elsewhere on the attributes of a surgeon. While the nature and scope of surgery have changed significantly since Ratten's time, the attributes of a surgeon remain largely similar. But it is unfair to compare a surgeon of yesteryear with a surgeon of today — the requirements and obligations are not the same. For example, the revered surgeon Weary Dunlop was wonderful as a war surgeon but concerned many with his surgery in a conventional hospital setting.

If you want to pick your surgeon, ask an anaesthetist. At the head of the operating table, they see more surgery than anyone else in the medical profession.

I commenced anaesthetic training some 60 years ago and I retired 20 years ago. If I were to be judged by today's standards, I would be severely criticised in light of the changes that have since occurred.

A century ago the number of operations performed per head of population was much lower and they carried a significant risk. Mortality was the benchmark.

Operations were performed by a general surgeon — there were no specialist surgeons as now, and surgery mostly involved trauma with fractures, wounds and the removal of lumps and bumps. Less frequently, they involved the opening of body cavities such as the abdomen, chest or head. Speed was necessary and was recognised as the mark of the successful surgeon.

Today the number and varieties of operations are dramatically different, as is the environment and social expectations in which the surgeon works. Mortality is extremely low and morbidity is the main issue.

The requirements, characteristics and requisites of a good surgeon include intellectual and technical skills, motivation — including persistence and a spirit of inquiry — judgement, self-discipline, integrity, humility, accountability, courage but not rashness, stamina — both physical and mental, power of prolonged concentration — and a sense of humour. A surgeon needs to accurately assess a situation and decide whether to operate or not, or to investigate further.

Temperament and personality are not felt to be critical and both introverts and extroverts can be equally successful today.

But what is a good surgeon? The answer comes down to the outcome of the surgery and the satisfaction of the patient — it is in the eye of the beholder. The outcome may be good, yet the patient is not satisfied; or the outcome may be bad yet the patient may be very satisfied. A good doctor in a patient's eye may not be a good doctor in medical eyes.

The outcome of surgery is not as easy to measure as it may appear and it is well recognised that the outcomes of large numbers of patients are required to determine any significant differences between surgeons' results.

It was well accepted that the greater the volume of work a surgeon does — within limits — the greater is their surgical experience and post-operative mortality is reduced. This is less so today because of newer surgical skills, laboratories and new teaching methods.

A good surgeon today has to be a good technician, a good communicator and a good team member, qualities not highly rated a hundred years ago.

A surgeon requires training, a knowledge of basic medical sciences and technological support, skilled anaesthesia and skilled assistants. But to be more certain of a good outcome you need good post-operative care. Surgeons should teach, publish and audit their work, and undertake research.

There are many sayings about surgeons. Here are just a few:

- A surgeon needs the heart of a lion, the eye of an eagle and the hands of a lady.

- Surgery is primarily a discipline not of the hand but of the mind and character.
- Anyone whose shape of hand and range of finger movements lies within normal limits can be taught and learn surgical procedures.
- The sensory sides of a surgeon's hands are more important than motor power. They feel.
- Hardly any temperament is a bar to a surgical career. They can be introvert or extrovert but having said that you can generally pick the surgeon.
- A surgeon is not born, and manual dexterity required to be a good surgeon can be learnt.
- As said by New York surgical teacher Dr Spencer '…it is all right for the patient to think you walk on water as long as you don t believe it.'

Ratten's surgical training

HOW COULD someone with no medical training or qualifications, and specifically no surgical training, achieve the skills that Ratten obviously had? He was a self-trained man and he must have been academically bright, technically gifted and possessed of the right kind of personality. If that reasoning is correct, there could be three stages to his training.

Prior to 1907 he had worked as a dentist in NSW and Queensland, and he had an uncle, Arthur Ratten, who had medical qualifications. It was also claimed, very doubtfully, that he had worked as a dresser at the Maryborough Hospital and had attended a dental mechanics course in Texas, America. Both would have assisted him in gaining basic medical understanding and the development of certain technical skills.

Between 1907 and 1914, as the medical practitioner in Sheffield, he observed and assisted medical practitioners at the Devon Hospital at Latrobe — Drs Ferris and Walpole — and practitioners at the Launceston General Hospital. Dr Ramsay provided Ratten with a glowing reference.

He reportedly practised surgery on rabbits and ewes, and it was jokingly said that there was not a rabbit left in Sheffield with an appendix. During World War I when he was on active service between October 1914 and March 1915, he was in Egypt and conceivably obtained some surgical experience, but that was before hostilities started there.

Ratten had his own hospital in Sheffield and provided the only surgical service in the region, including trauma which was important in a rural area.

From 1917 when he was appointed as surgeon superintendent he practised on the public.

He had a mentor in Dr MacGowan, who was said to be a good surgeon and had been responsible for suggesting Ratten's appointment to the Government. Ratten read widely and had an extensive collection of books including *Medical Clinics of North America, Medical Clinics of Chicago, Surgical Clinics of North America* and *Surgical Clinics of Chicago*.

In considering what surgical skills were required at the time it is necessary to understand that surgery was much more restricted in scope than it is today because of limited ability to diagnose problems, limited equipment, instruments and medication, a lack of trained anaesthetists and the absence of such things as blood transfusions. Expectations were much lower.

Most surgery was done by general practitioners and any practitioner who wanted to train and obtain a recognised specialist qualifications in surgery went overseas, usually to the United Kingdom.

There was no formal surgical training or qualification in Australia until the Royal Australasian College of Surgeons was established in 1928.

In Ratten's time surgical training was either through apprenticeship or else the surgeon was largely self-taught. It is jokingly said that surgical training in the past was largely a case of being shown how to do one operation, doing the second yourself and teaching on the next — see one, do one, teach one.

It is also said that when a new treatment was developed it was initially described as 'the best thing since the invention of sliced bread' but when complications resulted it was so bad that 'you wouldn't subject your mother-in-law to it'; finally, when the dust settled, the treatment found its true place in medicine.

Nothing is clear-cut in medicine and with the expansion of knowledge, views on acceptable standards are changing all the time.

Ratten's Ability as a Surgeon

TO properly assess Ratten's surgical ability the late Professor Rimmer advised me that a structural analysis was required; I have not done this, nor am I certain that it can be done because of the passage of time and the scarcity of documentation.

In assessing Ratten's surgical ability we need to consider the range and scope of his surgery, review his operation notes and statistics on his morbidity and mortality, compare his results with those of other centres, patient reports, medical practitioners' reports and his influence on surgery.

He was interested only in surgery, operating daily on an average of fifteen patients in a session; he was reluctant to attend outpatients.

The official number of operations performed in the hospital increased quite dramatically in the first few years Ratten was there because he changed the method of recording operations.

Previously it had been the number of patients operated on but now it was the number of procedures performed — a quite different statistic. A media report in 1925 said that since 1917 the number of operations performed each year increased from 700 to 3000.

The scope of Ratten's surgery was very wide and I have collated the following list from Professor Rimmer's book *A Portrait of a Hospital*, personal communications, *The Mercury* and other media, Royal Commissions, Inquiries and hospital records. The list includes appendicectomies, skin grafts, bone grafts, thyroidectomies, thyroid transplants, remaking of faces — I assume this to be plastic surgery — caesarean sections, bowel surgery and craniotomies.

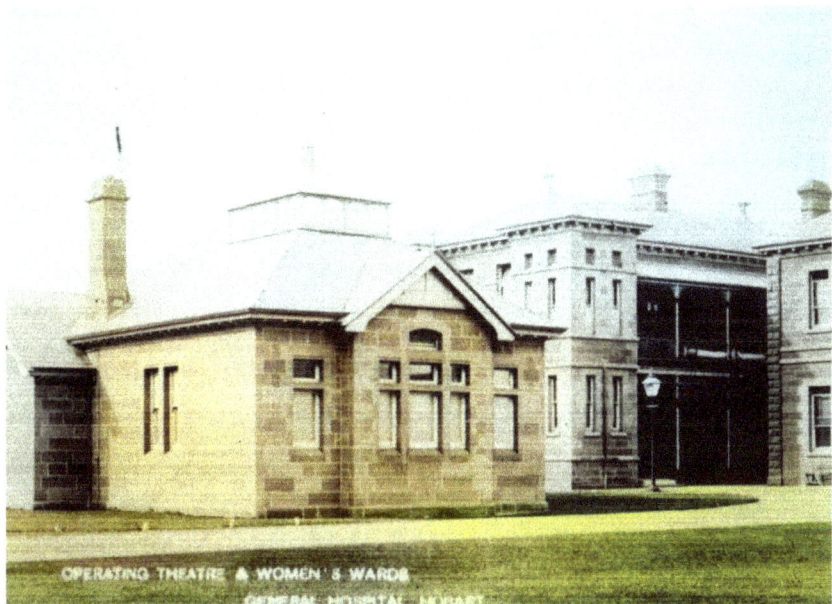

The operating theatre at the Hobart General Hospital in Ratten's day. It was separate from the main hospital building. There was no recovery room and patients were transferred straight from the theatre to the ward.

It is not possible to review his operation notes as they are not available. Many records were destroyed when the basement of the Royal Hobart Hospital was flooded in the 1970s.

Ratten was known for appendicectomies using a dexterous technique of rapid keyhole surgery. Medical practitioners still talk about the Ratten appendicectomy scar, which they say probably denoted the removal of a normal appendix — yet there are records of patients who had a Ratten appendicectomy still with their appendix. Prior to 1917 an appendicectomy took about an hour; this was reduced to 20 minutes after Ratten's arrival, and he had the time down to 10 minutes in 1923.

Statistics on morbidity are not available and statistics on mortality are very limited. In 1918 the mortality rate for surgical procedures at the Hobart General Hospital was recorded as 0.5 per cent, about 20 a year. In 1919-20 it rose to 0.8per cent but this is possibly explained by the increased scope of surgery in general. Another potential variable is the definition of mortality rate — is it a death in the operating theatre, a death occurring within 24 hours of an operation or even a death within 30 days of an operation? Without that information little comment can be made.

Regrettably, there is no data which allows a comparison of Ratten's surgical results with other centres.

He did not involve himself to any real extent in medical education other than that of resident medical officers and the occasional medical student from the mainland. He was not a member of the BMA, so he was not involved with their educational activities. He did communicate with interstate medical practitioners, so he would have kept up to date to a limited extent. He was not known to have attended conferences or gone overseas to gain further experience, as most leading medical practitioners did in those days. There is no evidence that he published in medical journals, but he used the *Mercury* to advantage. That was in complete contrast to the professional activities of leading surgeons such as Sir James Ramsay and Dr Sweetnam.

While little significance can be attached to patients' comments, they do give an insight as to how he was regarded. Many times when I have been giving my talk about Ratten I have been chided by elderly members of the audience about my implied criticism of Ratten and they have vocally defended him.

A collective view is more useful than individual opinions. Patients had confidence in him and grateful patients presented him with a testimonial (see next page) and a blackwood desk in 1921 after the Ratten Doubts Revocation Act had been passed and his position at the Hobart General Hospital as surgeon superintendent was secure. He was known as 'the people's doctor' and described as 'the wizard of the scalpel'. *(Truth* 7th July 1926)

It was said that patients were more impressed by the attention they received from Dr Ratten than from honorary doctors who visited the hospital in hours they could spare and that they received better care than in expensive private hospitals. As one critic said, 'These people didn't know what was good for them.'

Reports on Ratten's ability as a surgeon by his colleagues may be

Testimonial from Patients.

To Dr. Victor Ratten, Surgeon
Medical Superintendent of the Hobart General Hospital.

Sir,

HAVING been Patients for Special Surgical Operations, we take this opportunity of recording our confidence and gratitude for the good health enjoyed by us.

WE are pleased at your appointment as Superintendent of the Hobart General Hospital, and trust you may be long spared to be a benefit to sufferers in our midst.

WE beg you to accept the gift of a Blackwood Writing Cabinet.

We are, yours sincerely

G. H. GALLOP	H. RAYWOOD	H. W. GREEN	MRS. COX	MRS. ELI MIDSON
A. CAIRNDUFF	— CLARK	M. A. BRUCE	MRS. GEASON	MRS. SHARP
O. S. TYLER	R. HEWETT	R. WILLIAMS	MRS. E. M. HARRIS	MRS. GRANT
W. CONNOR	A. F. H.	J. HOGERTY	MRS. N. LAKIN	MRS. IKIN
J. A. LARGE	H. WATSON	F. SMITHIES	MRS. A. E. MORRISON	MRS. OWEN
E. A. BRANDON	ROY McVILLEY	A. WILSON	MRS. M. MORLEY	MRS. TURNER
J. JOHNSON	W. MAHER	F. J. CLARKE	MRS. E. WEIR	MRS. BACKHOUSE
W. J. CUMMINE	L. STEVENSON	W. MERPHITT	MRS. TAYLOR	MRS. ETHEL EATON
A FRIEND	G. GARTH	A FRIEND	MRS. E. M. NICHOLLS	MRS. RUSSELL
W. G. MILLER	H. CORDELL	GEO. JOHNSTON	MRS. R. SCHOLTZ	MRS. THORNTON
G. F. CANNOCK	A. W. PEGG	H. B. JACOBSON	MRS. ALF. SCHOLTZ	MRS. M. TAIT
R. GLOCK	G. TURNER	PERCY MORGAN	MRS. ALOMES	MRS. J. JOHNSON
M. C.	V. TRIFFET	— MANNING	MRS. McKEAN	MRS. C. ARNOL
T. G. HUME	G. F. TERRY	G. W. H. LUTTRELL	MRS. W. A. POWELL	MRS. J. CLARK
C. C. WATSON	M. P. PILCHER	J. NICOLSON	MRS. M. TABOR	MRS. N. LAKE
F. ARGEE	J. MOLLROSS	C. ARNOL	MRS. WADDERTON	MISS W. GUY
A. DOWDING	C. LOVELL	A. W. POULTON	MRS. A. JORDEN	MISS A. CURRIE
E. J. O'BRIEN	H. R. OAKLEY	R. CLAYTON	MRS. C. NASH	MISS R. C. COSSUM
J. BENGER	— McKENDRICK	— CRISP	MRS. J. BOWDEN	MISS L. TERRY
T. LARGE	R. WEST	— CAPSTICK	MRS. H. W. GREEN	MISS G. TERRY
W. BADNOCK	T. TERRY	R. ANDERSON	MRS. E. CLARKE	MISS B. GRAY
R. REDMAN	R. NEAVE	E. DWYER GRAY.	MRS. A. WILSON	MISS E. FORD
L. NEVELL	E. KERRISON	H. R. PEACOCK	MRS. D. MASON	MISS M. WILSON
H. HOPGOOD	W. FLEMING	FRIEND	MRS. W. MASON	MISS E. LORD
V. E. DENNING	C. SIMS	NAT. EDWARDS	MRS. M. JACKSON	MISS E. FORSYTHE
C. HARRISON	W. BELBIN	MASTER G. ARNOL	MRS. C. C. BRANWICK	MISS E. SEAGER
W. MUSK	J. R. LAZENBY	MASTER C. ARNOL	MRS. R. B. WOOD	MISS E. MANLEY
E. CARRICK	R. DODGE	MRS. J. NICOLSON	MRS. K. TURVEY	MISS H. SPOTSWOOD
E. LAMPKIN	C. M. BROWN	MRS. J. ANDERSON	MRS. G. WARNER	MISS C. M QUEENIE
— FITZGERALD	W. P. CHAPMAN	MRS. BENJAMIN	MRS. M. GREENLAND	MISS BING
P. LYNCH	T. R. CHANDLER	MRS. F. HARRIS	MRS. C. SUTCLIFFE	MISS M. EATON
J. MASON	W. RICHARDSON	MRS. W. WARNE	MRS. H. BARNES	MISS B. TAIT

" At even, ere the sun was set,
" The sick, O Lord, around Thee lay,
" O in what divers pains they met,
" O with what joy they went their way."

Arthur Dunning   Hon. Chairman

Geo H Gallop   Hon. Treasurer

Andrew Kirk   Hon. Secretary

considered biased, but there was at times a sneaking admiration of him as a doctor and of his surgical ability. Most doctors I have spoken with had never worked with Ratten but must have learned something from managing patients previously treated by him.

Some doctors, however, were not responsive to questions about Ratten. Dr Reg Lewis, the first specialist anaesthetist in Hobart in 1947, was a mentor of mine. He was a great racing enthusiast and lived opposite Barney Ratten in Sandy Bay. When questioned about Ratten he would deftly change the topic and avoid answering the question. Dr Jean Oakes was direct in her response and just said: 'Leave him alone'. Both were anaesthetists and possibly professionally and socially involved with him.

Sir Clifford Craig commented that Ratten had a very strong personality and extraordinary skill in handling patients and soliciting implicit trust; his standing was enhanced by a press hostile to the BMA and the attention that body paid to him. Sir William Crowther believed that the poorer people under Ratten and the present system received the best attention they could get anywhere.

Dr Goddard said Ratten was an extraordinary man and a remarkable technician, despite misgivings about his qualifications. Dr Goddard was one of the resident doctors who resigned from the Hobart General Hospital when Ratten was appointed surgeon superintendent in 1917.

Dr Franklyn Fay, son of Dr Frank Fay MC, who was largely responsible for negotiating the return of BMA to the Hospital in 1930, said Ratten was a danger in his early days for his poor judgment, but that by the end of his career he was a good operator. Roe recounts that Ratten was 'a super-heroic surgeon, and now, while draining of tubercular glands and sores continued, there also appeared pneumectomy (alias pneumomectomy, lung excision) and pneumonotomy (lung excision) the subjects perhaps being tubercular.'

Dr Hardy Wilson said Ratten left a legacy of the famous small right iliac fossa incision which became his trademark and which was supposed to be the result of the removal of a normal appendix. Dr Sam Murdock told me of one of his patients who had had a Ratten appendicectomy later had a barium enema which showed an appendix. Dr Chris Edwards operated on a Ratten patient who had an appendicectomy scar and still had an appendix. This is potentially extremely dangerous — it makes diagnosis difficult if the patient is seen for abdominal pain and say they have had an appendicectomy and a scar to prove it.

Dr Cam Duncan, the first pathologist appointed to the hospital, said that he arrived on 4th April 1936 and spent the next morning in the hospital watching the (in)famous Dr Ratten operating. He did about fifteen operations — mainly normal appendices through a one-inch incision— but there was one case that still sticks in his memory: a young woman three months pregnant who had a small dark 'ovarian cyst' which was removed. 'Not surprisingly, she aborted soon afterwards — but how could a newcomer like me tell him?'

Dr Des Cooper, a medical student from Melbourne in the 1940s, described how Ratten operated with his face mask off his nose, did not change his gown between operations and had all the instruments for the day put on a single table in the operating theatre. Dr Fay and Dr David Gibson confirmed this. This contrasts with Professor Rimmer's view that Ratten insisted upon an extremely high standard of hygiene. Rimmer also said that Ratten emphasised the need for teamwork and refused to operate with obsolete instruments.

Dr Lachlan Hardy Wilson was another medical student from Melbourne who spent time at the Royal Hobart Hospital. It was 1940 and he was a sixth year medical student. He was drafted to spend two weeks assisting Ratten every morning with his operating lists.

He said Ratten was a deft operator but clearly lacked any proper knowledge of pathology. It was the era of his famous gastro-jejunostomy operation which he did with considerable skill but whether the patients required such treatment or whether the result gave them any benefit is much less clear.

He described two deaths during those two weeks. One was due to the wartime shortage of anaesthetists; it was Ratten's habit to order the anaesthetist to start the next anaesthetic, ether in those days, saving him time between cases. On this occasion he was still completing the suturing of the gastro-jejunostomy. The theatre scout sister was absent. 'When we looked up the patient had gagged and was dead.'

The second case was even less impressive. It was a grossly fibrotic gall

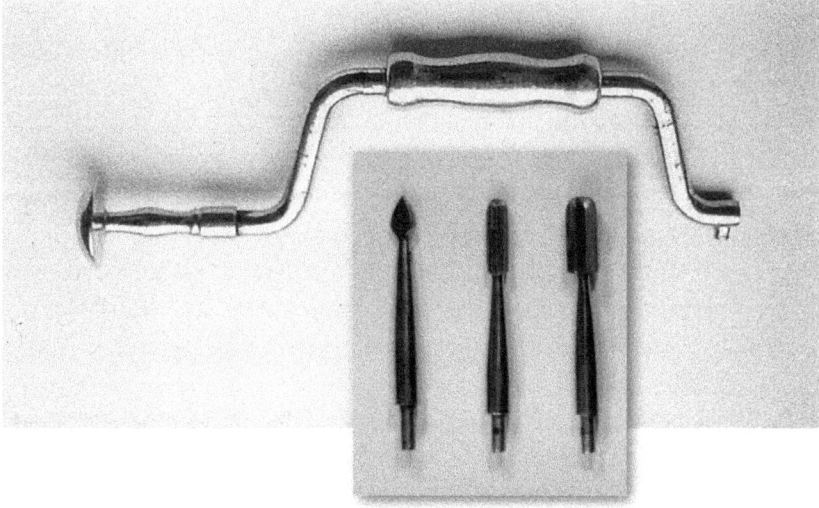

Among Ratten's instruments were these devices he used around 1940 for cerebral and spinal operations. Basically a nickel-plated brace and bit, the set consisted of a perforator (left in the lower image) with two burring bits. It was described by Professor Simpson as rather crudely made without any maker's name. The brace is engraved with the letters PHD.

bladder which the surgeon was unable to detach from the liver. He did a rough sort of clawing removal, stuffed the incision with packs and sent the patient back to the ward where she very promptly died.

In other areas he dabbled with laminectomies, an incision into the backbone to obtain access to the spinal cord, some of which were described as disastrous.

And yet the public adored him and his colleagues were forced to put up with his extraordinary hospital contract. This, it was said, was the lever to get him out of the position of surgeon superintendent. It involved operating five mornings a week and no other duties that Dr Wilson could remember as being required.

Professor Donald Simpson, an eminent neurosurgeon from Adelaide, said he was a visiting medical student in 1946. He said that Ratten was no longer surgeon superintendent but was still very much part of the local medical scene.

He was told that Ratten had performed a number of brain and

spinal operations and had pioneered surgery for hydrocephalus, using gold tubes to drain the spinal fluid into some unspecified cavity. A media report in 1925 said that 38 babies had been saved from death by cranial operations.

Ratten was also said to have pioneered bowel surgery in Hobart. Dr John Hunn said some of this involved bowel anastomosis; this is where bowel is joined together for particular problems. Sometimes Ratten did the anastomosis the wrong way around and patients were often sent to Sir Hugh Devine the expert in Melbourne for corrective surgery. The operation became known as 'derattenisation'.

Another operation Ratten did frequently was thyroidectomy, often for overactive thyroid glands — thyrotoxicosis. The recognised treatment was preparation with iodine before surgery to prevent post-operative problems. Ratten neglected to do this, and his mortality rate was 5 per cent. A recognised complication with this operation is damage to the recurrent laryngeal nerve, which if damaged results in hoarseness and other problems. Ratten had a very high incidence of this complication and Dr Roger Connolly had the statistics for this — another casualty of records lost in a hospital flood. Dr Nigel Abbott said Ratten was still using chloroform for this operation, which was considered dangerous.

Ratten could be very convincing and not always to the patient's advantage. Dr Fay saw a patient who explained that she had seen Ratten, who had diagnosed carcinoma of the cervix and recommended surgery. After examining the woman, Dr Fay said 'I believe you have a cervical erosion but perhaps it is best if you see a Melbourne specialist.' The woman did and she was advised that surgery was unnecessary.

Some time later he again saw the patient, who had had a hysterectomy by Ratten. When he asked her about it she replied, 'Well, Dr Ratten said he could cure me, and I felt I should take the safest course'.

Dr Heather Gibson grew up in Tasmania and was aware of some of Ratten's background. She was a resident at the Royal Hobart Hospital from 1942-45. At the time Dr J B Muir was surgeon superintendent, and the other staff member was Dr Stymie Gaha. She said Ratten did not do much at the hospital other then operate — no outpatients, no ward rounds and one weekend on call in three. She had to assist him at operations. There was no routine preparation of patients for surgery and Ratten sent his own patients to the hospital for operation the next day. While his skills were good, she felt that he did not know what he was doing or forgot to do what he had intended; his gauge of a good operation was its brevity and the neatness of the scar.

She can recall a few disasters, including an infant dying from intussusception (a serious condition in which part of the intestine slides into an adjacent part, which often blocks food or fluid from passing through) and a tibial osteotomy to cure a bow leg resulting in osteomyelitis.

Ratten did not attempt to teach the residents and they did not like working with him. He was described as bombastic — if something didn't go well it was 'Just bad luck,' 'No-one could have done better,' or 'I have done my best and now it is up to the nursing staff.' That is, others took the rap if it didn't go well. This is no different to what still happens today when after an operation a surgeon says to a patient who has non-specific issues following surgery that it must be the anaesthetic. It must also be remembered that this was during the war and Ratten was nearing the end of his career.

Dr Gibson was never aware that Ratten had any physical handicaps or an injured shoulder. She recalls one Saturday night when, called back to the hospital, he had wads of money stuffed into his operating suit pockets so no one could take it. Was that the results of his day's gambling at the races?

It is difficult to determine Ratten's influence on surgery and surgical education. From what has been said, Ratten lacked judgment; he did operations others would not do; he experimented and dabbled. Not unusual, perhaps, and that is how medicine progresses, but it is not done in isolation and without peer support.

He prevented and actively opposed the involvement of other doctors and it seems he operated at times for his own benefit. His work was not audited, not presented at medical meetings and nor was it published — all the normal ways to compare results with others and share knowledge. A different explanation is offered by Dr Peter Braithwaite: 'It is understandable that as a practicising surgeon he didn't publish. You have to have something to say, not something everyone already knows.' Ratten opposed increases in hospital staff — in effect, opposing medical progress.

This was at a time of change in medicine with more specialties coming to be formally recognised: in 1928 The Royal Australasian College of Surgeons; in 1929 the British College of Obstetrics and Gynaecology; in 1930 the Association of Physicians of Australasia; in 1934 the Australian Society of Anaesthetists; in 1935 the Australian and New Zealand Association of Radiology.

All of these organisations evolved to establish colleges in their specialities in both Australia and New Zealand and have received Royal assent.

One final example of Ratten's work: occasionally he would do an operation called a mastoidectomy, an operation for a chronic infection behind the ear. Reputedly, all of Ratten's mastoidectomy patients died. Today it would be done by an ear, nose and throat (ENT) specialist. After the arrival of such a surgeon in the hospital, patients started surviving. In a bitter irony, Ratten's son, Wing Commander John Ratten, had a mastoidectomy in 1945 in England from which he did not recover.

Ratten's duties as Surgeon Superintendent

Some insight into Ratten's view of his own capacity as a surgeon can be gained from the duties he contracted to undertake at the Hospital. They are evidence of overconfidence and this onerous workload goes some way to explain why he was often criticised for neglect of duty — it would hardly have been possible for a single doctor to successfully fulfill everything in such a schedule. Added to this was his unreasonable opposition to staff increases, which could have alleviated some of the strain.

An incomplete list of his duties includes:

▌ Examination of day cases and sick patients before operating.
▌ A full round in each ward daily.
▌ Operating from 9am to 1pm and often longer.
▌ All urgent operations at any time of day or night.
▌ Examination of sick nurses and their treatment.
▌ Consultations with resident staff.
▌ Removal of all sutures.

▌Signing all requisitions, diet cards etc.

▌Outpatients every 2pm Tuesday and Thursday, seldom finishing before 4pm.

▌Lecturing surgical classes every Thursday night for one hour.

▌Committee meetings every Wednesday.

▌Board meetings once a month, and often special meetings.

▌Medical cases especially asking for Dr Ratten for examination and treatment — this could be as many as 75 patients.

▌Setting of most fractures.

▌Appointments with pharmaceutical travellers.

▌Attending nearly all serious casualties.

▌Conferences with heads of Medical, Secretarial and other departments.

▌Post-mortem examinations.

▌Available on telephone every minute of the 24 hours.

▌All correspondence on enquiries for operations, patients' conditions, certificates etc. every day.

An overly ambitious and power-hungry person may promise to shoulder such an impossible amount of work to gain favour and appear to be indispensable, especially if there are concealed issues with their qualifications and professional history.

So after nineteen years of work as surgeon superintendent and all the controversy and contention that marked his career, this cavalier promise to perform the impossible is one principal reason why Ratten left no enduring surgical legacy.

The Royal Australasian College of Surgeons

THE ROYAL AUSTRALASIAN COLLEGE OF SURGEONS was established in 1928 and became the standard setting, training and examining body for the specialty of surgery, granting Fellowship of the Royal Australasian College of Surgeons (FRACS).

It does raise the question as to whether Ratten in any way had any influence on the establishment of the RACS or whether they considered him in any way in their deliberations.

Australia was a century behind England in establishing a college of surgeons. In 1800 the Royal College of Surgeons of London was incorporated, and they awarded an undergraduate qualification, Member of the Royal College of Surgeons (MRCS). In 1834 they awarded a postgraduate diploma for specialist surgeons, Fellow of the Royal College of Surgeons (FRCS).

On 19th November 1925 Drs Syme, Hamilton, Russell and Devine wrote to senior surgeons in the clinical schools of Australasia and this letter is the foundation stone of the Royal Australasian College of Surgeons. The letter expresses concerns which could relate to Ratten:

'Senior surgeons and surgical specialists in all States of Australia have noticed with much concern a growing disregard by younger practitioners of recognised ethics of surgical practice combined with a spirit of commercialism tending to degrade the high traditions of the surgical profession.

'Difficult and dangerous surgical operations are undertaken by practitioners who have not been properly trained in surgical principles

and practice and who divide fees with colleagues who refer the patients to them. *They also operate in small and inadequately equipped
hospitals which have recently sprung into existence in large numbers.
The public has no means of judging the competency of these so-called
surgeons and surgical specialists and the efficiency of these hospitals.
It is felt that steps should be taken to counteract these conditions.'*

The only unambiguous reference to Ratten in College records is the
stenographic record of proceedings of the first Annual General Meeting
on 2nd April 1928 in the Albert Hall, Canberra during discussion following reading of a paper on hospitals and hospital methods.

Dr Sweetnam, who had been Surgeon Superintendent at the Launceston General Hospital, addressed the meeting on the situation at the Hobart General Hospital:

*'We have in the hospital a man who is not qualified and he was put
there by the Government and they passed a special act of parliament
to allow him to practise. We cannot shift him. There are no facilities
for surgical experience — they operate in private hospitals, and you
know what that means. It never leads anywhere. Anything we try to
do to alter the position is interpreted by the public as jealously. The
position is absolutely hopeless as far as a body go in altering the conditions and I can see no way out of the position at all except by the
death of that man.*

*'He is stuck there, and he cannot practise anywhere else in Austral-
asia. He will stick there unless he is driven out. I can see no body who
could function better in that capacity than the College of Surgeons
and I put it forward as a suggestion to the Council of this College
that they seriously consider the advisability of communicating with
the Government and pointing out to them the serious condition of
affairs that are existing and I would like this council to very seriously
consider the advisability of doing something in that direction.*

*'That point is so very very important that my colleagues in Tasma-
nia thought it would be a very excellent chance for me to bring before
this college the advisability of perhaps doing something. He is appointed for a period of three years at a time. I think his appointment is up
in 14 months' time. If anything is done by this College, it will have to*

be done within the next year and details of what the College could do will be readily supplied by the Tasmanian Doctors if the Council would consider the matter at all'.

The Council decided not to publish the discussion on the hospital question at the AGM in Canberra because it might be dangerous for the speakers if it were published.

I have no knowledge if the RACS involved itself in the Ratten dispute, either officially or unofficially.

There were 41 Founders of the RACS including two Tasmanians — David Henry Edward Lines and Sir John Ramsay. Of the 165 Foundation Fellows of the RACS, there were again two Tasmanians — Gustav Heinz Hogg and John Stoddart Barr.

Ratten as a Person

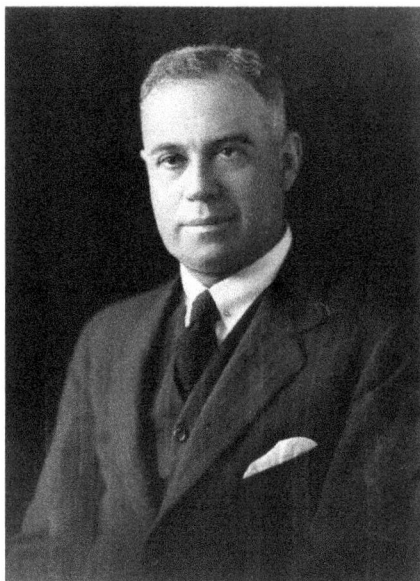

AUTHOR'S COLLECTION

RATTEN was something of a diplomat — skilled in manipulation, fond of back-door deals and with a talent for strategic alliances. He ignored situations and hoped they would go away. He did not dispute what was said against him and never spoke publicly against his detractors. If cornered, he would call for an inquiry and hope his friends would help him out.

He was not a big man, though a bit stout — 5ft 8in (173cm), 12st 4lbs (78kg), chest measurement 33-38in (84-97cm), with good eyesight at the time of enlistment in the army.

Quietly spoken but with a gravelly voice, he was always somewhat flamboyant and trendy; when it was normal for a male to be bearded, he was clean-shaven, wore pinstripe suits, smoked cigars, loved cars and drove a Rolls-Royce. He was a determined character, as evidenced by how he negotiated his registration as a dentist in Queensland, obtaining his American medical qualification and fighting the BMA.

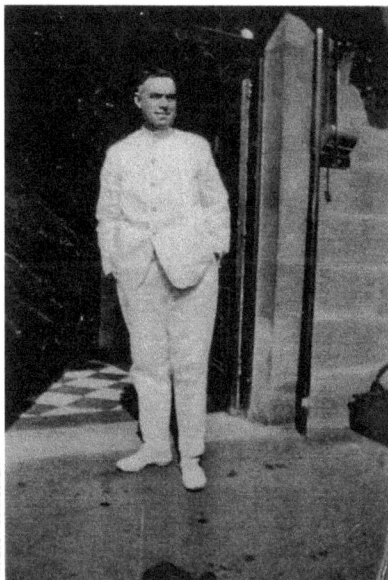

AUTHOR'S COLLECTION

He was somewhat arrogant, a quality common among surgeons in days gone by. If an operation did not go well, he blamed someone else. He would say to the patient or the relative that he had done his best and that now it was up to the resident or the nursing staff.

When discussing his needs with the Hospital Board he said that he required 200 of the hospital beds 'because the public wants me'. The total number of beds in 1925 was 250.

He was aggressive in his work and would have been seen by some as irresponsible. But it must be acknowledged that progress in medicine often requires a medical practitioner to take risks — these days such risks are mitigated by ethics committees and the like. He was in Sheffield when there was an appendectomy epidemic, and he performed surgery others would not attempt.

He did not consult local doctors, even those recognised as having great experience; instead he sought advice outside the State and sent some of his pathological specimens elsewhere. This perhaps explains amendments made to the Medical Act, which required a medical practitioner to see a colleague if requested.

He was helpful to private practitioners — obviously his source of referral— and provided them promptly with letters after seeing patients.

He could be forgiving and showed a soft streak; a resident spoke of Ratten as 'Rats' in front of a patient. The patient repeated this to Ratten but he forgave the resident. He was seen to break down crying when he had to explain to an eminent local identity that they had terminal cancer. He named one of his racehorses after his deceased son.

He was socially inclined: a member of the Athenaeum Club, the Naval and Military Club, the Returned Sailors and Soldiers Imperial League of Australia Club (RSSILA), now the RSL, the Tasmanian Automobile

Club, The Royal Yacht Club of Tasmania, the Masonic Society and a life member of the Tasmanian Racing Club. But he never joined any medical organisations.

In Sheffield he became involved in several sporting organisations and was noted for his love of gambling. He challenged locals to billiards matches and pigeon shooting contests, reputedly for high stakes.

Ratten knew how to be a good boss and looked after his staff at the Hobart General Hospital, particularly the nurses, but this created difficulties when he interfered with the matron's disciplinary powers. He wanted his own personal theatre nursing staff. He gave his staff signed photographs and ensured that amenities were adequate, suggesting to the Board that a tennis court be built 'for their health, amusement recreation and to promote happiness'.

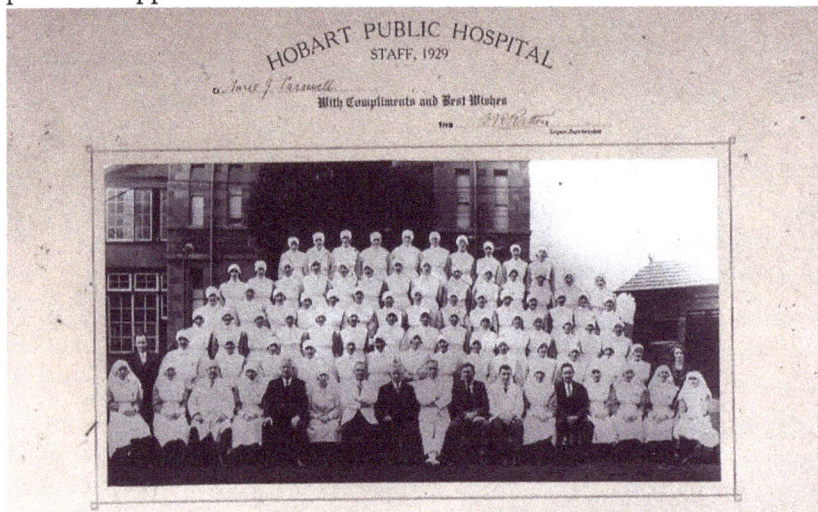

HOBART PUBLIC HOSPITAL STAFF, 1929

Ratten knew how to cultivate friends in high places and on all sides of politics. When Governor Sir Harry Barron visited Sheffield, he got the train to Railton and Ratten drove him to Sheffield. The American Consul, Mr H D Baker, was Ratten's guest in Sheffield for a few days in 1909. Premier Lee from the same electorate of Wilmot appointed Ratten as surgeon superintendent. Ogilvie, a lifelong friend and supporter, protected him in many ways and drafted the Ratten Doubts Act; Ogilvie's wife was a member of the Hospital Board. Justice Ewing, who conducted the 1918

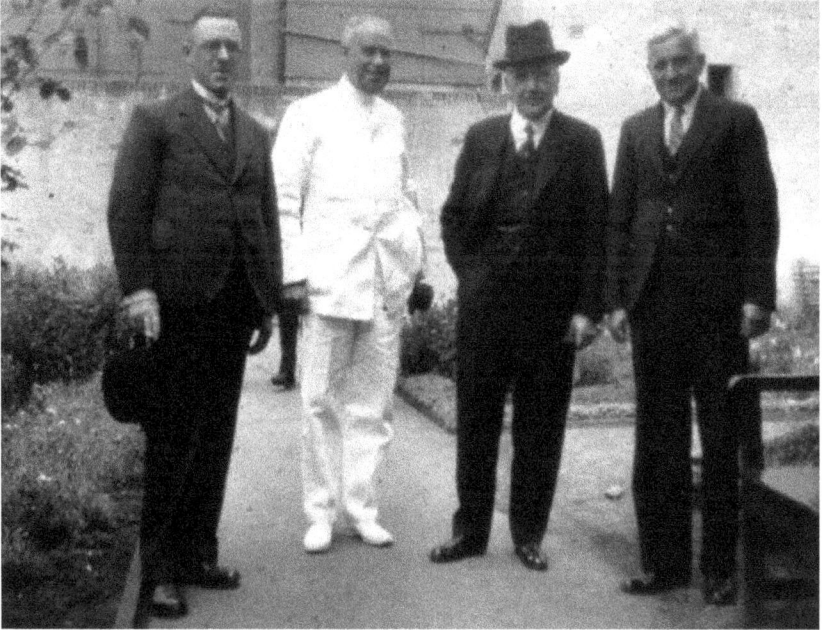

Ratten moved in high circles. Here he is with (left to right) Albert Ogilvie, Premier of Tasmania 1934-1939; Ratten; Sir Ernest Clark, Governor of Tasmania 1933-1945; and H R Baker, Chairman of Hobart Public Hospital

Royal commission, was a friend. Through these friendships he was protected and was even promised a seat on the Medical Council of Tasmania, which never eventuated. Dr Gaha and Dr Carruthers, two of his supporters, became Minister for Health and Director of Public Health and Chairman of the Hospital Board respectively. The Government bought Ratten's St Helens Hospital.

In 1948 Ratten was an independent candidate for the Tasmanian House of Assembly in the seat of Denison. His advertisement read:

'None better to express a real and practical health policy to Parliament. He will seek to express the will of the people — not the discussion of hidden and invisible forces. A real independent'.

Among the candidates were several who had drifted from the Labor ranks, unable to see eye-to-eye with the party. Ratten was for many years a member of the Labor Party and there was a move to offer him endorsement after the candidates had been chosen.

He had banners which read:
'If you can trust me with your life you can trust me with your vote.
Thousands of people have trusted me all their lives — you can trust
me with your vote.'
He was not elected.

It is said that Ratten never spoke publicly against his detractors but he did move against those who opposed him in the workplace, as evidenced by his dismissal of Dr Clark as previously outlined, and he actively opposed Dr Fay who was negotiating the return of the BMA to the hospital. His opposition often took the form of briefing local newspapers rather than talking directly to the hospital or the BMA. He had running battles with Matron Wade and after some years achieved her dismissal.

Ratten's greatest supporters were his patients, and he cultivated them. He knew how to get their confidence and their implicit trust.

And it wasn't only his patients he cultivated. My aunt's mother worked at the front desk of the Brisbane Hotel in Hobart and Ratten gave her boxes of chocolates.

He had business interests; he owned St Helens Hospital and was the principal shareholder in Catamaran Coal, an ownership which got him into significant trouble.

It must be said that he was dishonest, perhaps even a downright liar, perhaps even criminal. There is obviously the matter of his medical qualifications but there are several other examples. If he was an inveterate liar, did he lie to his patients?

In 1907 when he returned from America, he said at an interview that he had undertaken four years of study in America and repeated it again in a statutory declaration when he registered as a medical practitioner in South Australia.

On another occasion he said he had undertaken three years as a medical student in Australia — which he had not — and in 1914 he was elected a Fellow of the Royal Institute of Public Health in London on the basis of his bogus medical qualification.

He obtained a Bachelor of Science in 1929 from the Intercollegiate University of Chicago — see next page. No record of this institution can be found, and he was living in Tasmania at the time.

He had given his qualification in *Who's Who* as MD (Tas). No such qualification existed at the time, and that the Government had conferred such a qualification on him was a falsehood that persisted until recent times.

As previously noted, he received a life suspension for race fixing and was in trouble with the Betting Control Board and with the Hospital Board for supplying Catamaran coal to the hospital.

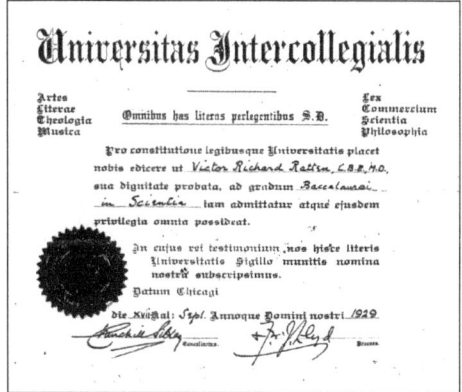

Universitas Intercollegialis

RATTEN, Victor Richard, C.B.E., M.D. (Tas.): son of Rev. G. W. Ratten of Melb.; b. 1878; ed. Chicago Univ., U.S.A.; M.D. 1907; Surgeon Supt. Hobart Public Hosp.; served Gt. War, A.I.F. 1914-19, R.M.O. 12th Battn.; C.B.E. 1925; address, 50 Liverpool St., Hobart, Tas.

Radium went missing several times at the Hobart General Hospital and it was suggested that Ratten was using this very expensive substance on his private patients.

He raised private fees with his scam involving Gaha and was in difficulty with the taxation department — but perhaps that was viewed as a badge of honour.

Ratten was devious; he manipulated things to his advantage and for his whole time as surgeon superintendent be abused his right to private consultations and to private practice. It was never clearly defined, so he could interpret it however he wished and possibly he and the Board wanted to keep it that way. He would see a patient whom he would then send to Gaha who, without performing any sort of examination, would refer the patient back to Ratten, who could then charge a fee of one guinea.

Ratten's personal life has raised many questions. The matron at his hospital in Sheffield had a child whose father has never been named. Later in life the family suggested that a DNA test be undertaken; this was discouraged. He was known for bottom-pinching: one nurse said 'He pinched my sister's bottom but not mine — she was good-looking'. Reputedly he did not get on with his elder son John, but it is noted that when John was dying in England in 1945 Ratten set off there but only got as far as Colombo, turning back when he heard John had died.

While employed as surgeon superintendent Ratten was provided with quarters, light and fuel at the hospital and later maintained a residence at 167 Macquarie Street, now the site of the Downtowner hotel.

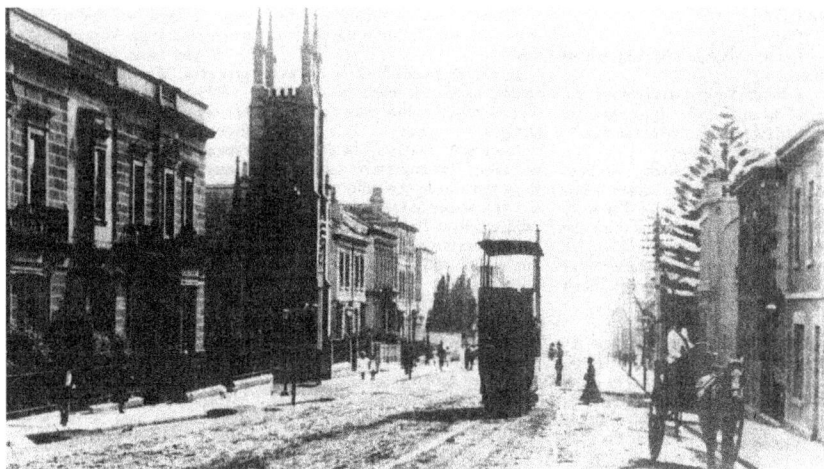

Ratten's mansion, 'Lalla Rookh,' 167 Macquarie Street, Hobart, at left.

Ratten separated from his wife in midlife, and she went to live in Sandy Bay. He was known for his philandering ways, his Rolls-Royce, his fast river launch and his lady friends. One was Dr Ethel Davis, a resident medical officer at the Hobart General Hospital. On one occasion the Hospital Board approved leave so they could go on holidays together. Ratten was accused of bringing a nurse back to the nursing home late one night.

When Ratten resigned as Surgeon Superintendent in 1936 Dr Davis left the hospital, remained his anaesthetist in private practice and looked after him in his old age.

Was Ratten a romantic? His house in Macquarie Street was named Lalla Rookh after an oriental romance by Irish poet Thomas Moore, published in 1817. He kept a framed photograph of Edith Cavell, the English nurse who helped Allied soldiers escape from German-occupied Belgium during World War I and was executed in 1915.

He had a 62ft (19-metre) luxury motor cruiser named *J'Attendrai,* a converted naval torpedo recovery craft.

Ratten had an innate talent for publicity and it is easy to say he was always seeking self-promotion. There was no television and only limited radio, so newspapers were how people learnt about local affairs and Ratten used them when it suited his purposes. On more than one occasion the hospital board had to instruct Ratten to send reports they required to them and not to the papers.

In 1938 on a radio program he was asked his opinion on an operation performed by an English doctor on a girl who had been 'criminally assaulted' — an abortion. He said some useful law might be passed to approve abortion to save life and health on a proper footing and suggested that abortion required the support of two medical practitioners and be referred to the police. Terms used then seem odd today — terms such as a 'certain event', 'criminally tampered with' and 'criminally assaulted'.

Ratten was associated with abortions at Highfield Hospital in Hobart and Gaha had been accused of performing a confidential operation on a nurse.

In December 1941 there was a report of the sudden death of a woman in hospital from peritonitis. It was due to internal perforation by an instrument but there was no evidence as to when, how or by whom the perforation was effected. The patient had asked to be operated on by Ratten and Gaha.

Ratten received many awards. He was recommended for and awarded the CBE (Commander of the British Empire) on the King's Birthday in 1925. He had previously been recommended in the 1924 King's Birthday and 1925 New Year's honours.

The citation read:

> 'Dr Victor Richard Ratten has rendered very eminent public service in his capacity of surgeon superintendent of the Hobart public hospital. Grave difficulties at one time arose between the Hospital board and medical practitioners and while it is not desirable at the present to review the causes of the dispute it is fitting to record the fact that the sick and suffering inmates of the hospital would have been left in a most critical position had Dr Ratten not remained loyal to the hospital board. His achievements as a surgeon have gained for him a very high place indeed in public estimation and it is largely due to

his skill and unremitting attention to his professional work that the Hobart public hospital has gained a very high place among similar institutions in Australia. The board of the hospital on many occasions have brought to the notice of the government their appreciation of Dr Ratten's services to the hospital'.

The following words were found added to the citation in another document. An 'afterthought' or a suggested afterthought?

'...and the government of the day accordingly considers that it is but fitting to commend Dr Ratten for some recognition'.

He was recommended for knight bachelor (KB) on three occasions, 1927,1939 and 1946, but it was not awarded. Dr John Ramsay was awarded the KB in 1927.

Ratten received the Silver Jubilee Medal in 1935, as did Mrs Ratten, Mrs Ogilvie, wife of Premier Ogilvie, Dr Ethel Davis and Dr Gaha.

Buckingham Palace. 'By command of his majesty the King the accompanying medal is forwarded to Dr V R Ratten CBE to be worn in commemoration of Their Majesties Silver Jubilee 6 May 1935'.

In 1936 he received the Coronation Medal.

Ratten's Cars

Much has been written about the cars of his early years, but his interest never waned and he drove a Rolls-Royce in the end. In the early days cars were a novelty but general interest in cars faded as they became more common. Ratten had cars in Brisbane when he was a dentist there, but the makes are not known. At outdoor social functions he would offer his car for fundraising activities.

Initially cars were novelties and at Sheffield School there was great excitement when somebody called 'Car coming!' and everybody would rush to the front fence to see this 'novel monster' go by.

On 31st January 1908 it was reported that he was shipping his 15hp four-cylinder Ford to Tasmania and by 1909 he had a 20hp four-cylinder Napier which was said to be very handsome and capable of a fair speed. It soon became obvious that since there were no Napier agents in the locality the car would have to be towed if there was a problem. By a horse, perhaps?

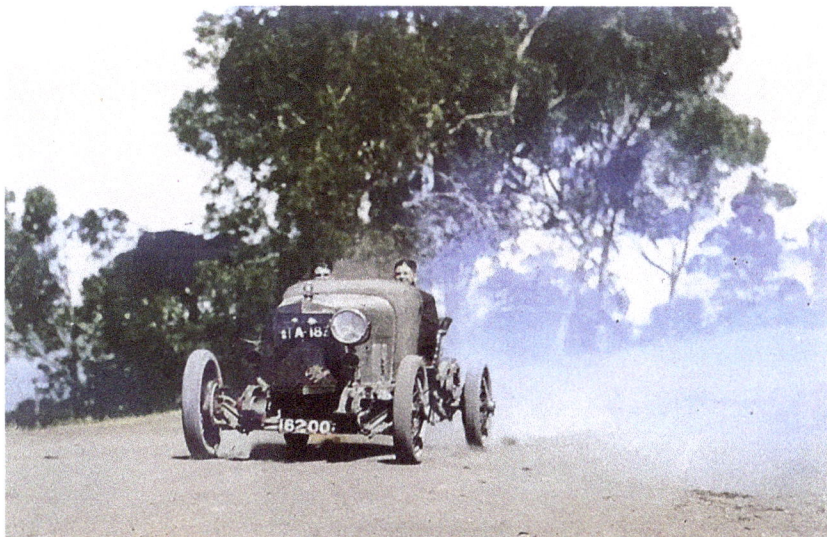

From a photograph found among Ratten's papers
— the car is thought to be a Napier

It is said he set records for travel from Sheffield to other parts of the district. By 1914 he had progressed to a single-seater, one of the most expensive cars yet imported into the commonwealth — a 33hp Fiat Lorraine Dietrich, painted silver and shaped like a bullet, pointed at both ends. It was a hill climb winner and was known locally as 'the Beetle'. Ratten had it modified to make the back dickey seat open flat to take an improvised stretcher. Fuel was gravity fed and to climb the steeper hills it was necessary to drive up in reverse.

He had his car problems, though — he was fined 2s 6d and half costs for exceeding the speed limit but that was not nearly as expensive as his collision with a cow, which cost him £30 in damage to the car.

A car certainly assisted Ratten more than a horse to get to accidents but it brought demands from him for bridges to be modified, which did not go down well with local authorities.

Clues as to his later cars can be gleaned from advertisements: 'Lost – Hudson wheel cap. Reward.' and 'Lost — three Packard car keys on ring'.

The Motor Vehicles and Traffic Act was passed in 1907 and required that every vehicle to be registered, fees paid for registration and a number assigned to the vehicle with plates supplied by the Registrar of Motor vehicles affixed to the vehicle. A list of those who had registered motor vehicles or motorcycles appeared in the *Police Gazette* on 26th March 1909. Ratten's number plate was 117 MV.

Ratten on the Turf

RATTEN HAD a lifelong interest in horses and horse racing. The first reference I have of this is his purchase of a racehorse in Brisbane in 1905 at a time when he was running his successful dental practice. The next reference is by Robson

'Horse racing continued in the pattern established from the first years of Van Diemen's Land when a dispute arose concerning whether a horse had been permitted to run on its merits; Dr Victor R Ratten in 1911 appealed against a decision by the Tasmanian Turf Club to disqualify him for life concerning the pulling of a racehorse'.

A jockey made a somewhat complicated complaint that Ratten had deliberately misrepresented a written message from the owner of the horse he was about to ride. Ratten had a horse in the race and the written message was to the effect that he thought the horse was a certainty and how he wanted him to race. Ratten did not give him the written message but said that the owner did not want him to win, that he should stop the horse as he was backing another horse, and that the owner would pay him a winning ride plus a few pounds extra. Ironically, the jockey's horse won.

An inquiry was initiated by the stewards of Newnham Racing Club, and it held two in camera sittings lasting eighteen hours. He was found guilty of attempting corrupt and fraudulent practices at Mowbray races. He appealed to the Tasmanian Turf Club, but the appeal was dismissed.

Ratten said he would appeal to the Supreme Court but he never did. Some time later it was reported that all reference to this affair had been

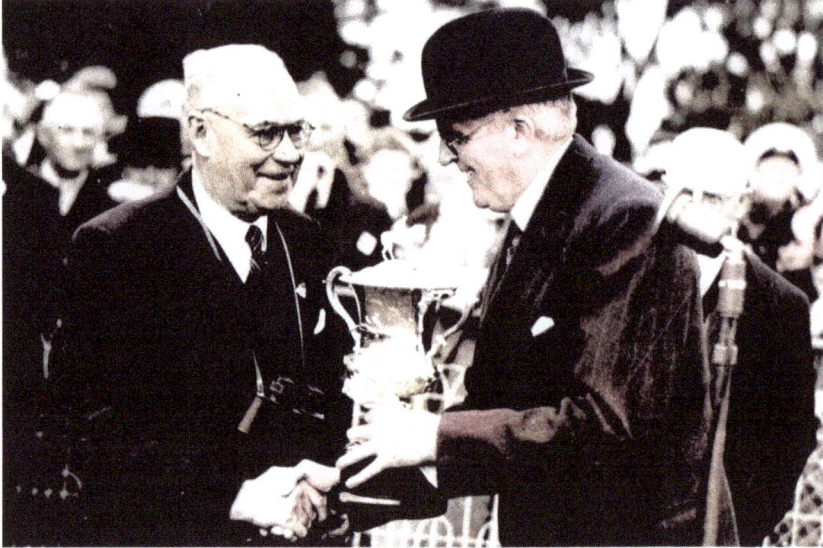

The Governor of Tasmania, Admiral Sir Hugh Binney, presents the 1947 Hobart Cup trophy to Victor Ratten

expunged from the minutes and this explains why there had been no Supreme Court action. The stewards also decided to forward a complaint to the Law Society regarding the action of a certain solicitor for a breach of professional etiquette. His disgrace was not confined to Tasmania; the *Truth* newspaper in Brisbane reported: 'Rotten Ratten. The disqualified doctor. Tasmanian Racing Scandal'.

These were interesting times and the use of pseudonyms by owners to conceal their identity was common from the earliest days right up to the present century after which it was prohibited. Ratten was in partnership with R (Dick) Page as 'Mr P Gare'. Betting was not like it is today, and a past secretary of the TRC once told me about a well-known personality, saying 'hold the race, I haven't got my money on yet — are they trying today?'

On one occasion there was an outburst from punters when a favourite owned by Ratten dwelt at the barrier. The starter was abused, and insults were hurled at Ratten.

After World War II Ratten emerged as a prominent owner. He won three consecutive Hobart Cups, an achievement since unmatched.

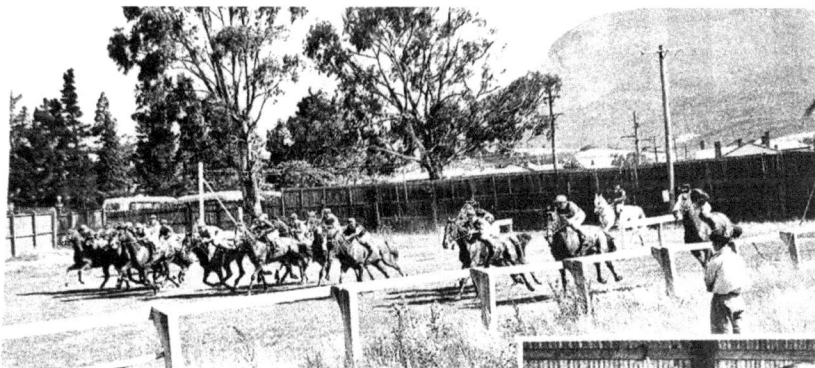

A race and course record was set in the running of the 1949 Hobart Cup, which was won by The Artist (owned by Dr V.R. Ratten, trained by C. Crossin and ridden by T. Unkovich). These Mercury archive images show the start (above), the cup presentation, the jockey weighing in and the winner getting a manicure.

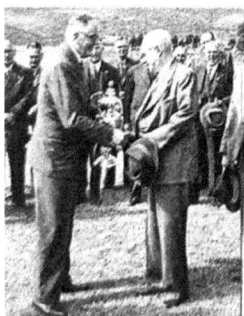

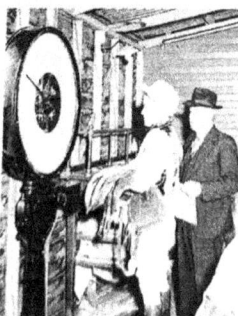

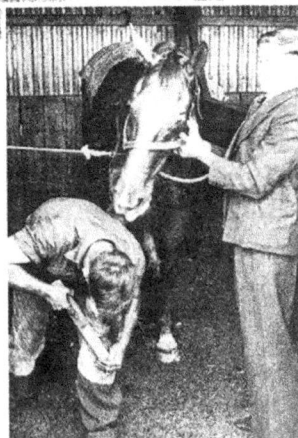

The caption reads:
A race and course record was set in the running of the 1949 Hobart Cup, which was won by The Artist (owned by Dr V. R. Ratten, trained by C. Crossin and ridden by T. Unkovich). These Mercury *archive images show the start (above), the cup presentation, the jockey weighing in and the winner getting a manicure.*

In 1947 he won with Wingfire, which he bought for 1000 guineas at the Melbourne sales. Wingfire was named in commemoration of his son John — 'Wing' came from Wing Commander and 'fire' from the Spitfire John flew. He had hoped to name the horse Spitfire — this was refused — and then tried Shangri-la, the name of John's spitfire, but that too was not available.

In 1948 he won with Evade which he owned in partnership with 'Mr P Gare' and in 1949 with The Artist which was owned solely by Ratten.

The winning cups were all sold at Barney Ratten's posthumous auction and are now in the in the Tasmanian Racing Club museum. At one time they were on display in the fashion window of a leading Hobart store.

All horses were mainland purchases, and all were trained by Cecil Crossin. Ratten's brother Frederick would pick the horses out and buy them for Ratten They were all foaled in the same year, 1941, and mainland jockeys were brought in for all the Cup winners. Scobie Breasley was the jockey in 1947.

Wingfire was the only one that was reasonably successful at stud in the Deloraine area. Ratten's horses won many other important races, including the Launceston Cup, the Doncaster Cup, the Tasmanian Guineas and the Newnham Cup. He was the leading owner in 1949.

Ratten was popular with racegoers but even more popular with jockeys because of his generosity. He took horses to race in Victoria and was the first to fly a horse to Melbourne.

He was quite a punter and spent some thousands of pounds each month, but it is not possible to confirm any figures. After a race meeting, he would count his winnings with his brother Frederick and his partner Dr Ethel Davis on his kitchen table. This was too much temptation for one of his housemaids who was charged and convicted of stealing £1370. She found the key to the safe under the pillow of his partner. A similar theft had occurred earlier when he was in Sheffield.

In 1952 he was in trouble with the betting control board and in response to a question said that he was 'almost quite sure'.

A horse, Paramente, its owner and trainer were banned for life in Tasmania when they refused a swab after coming fourth in a race. They said they would agree if the winner, Ratten's horse, The Artist, was also swabbed.

He was a prominent member of the racing fraternity and was a Tasmanian Amateur Jockey Club (TAJC) committee member for 20 years until 1947, then a committee member of the Tasmanian Racing Club (TRC) from 1947 to 1961, when he retired. He was made a life member.

Ratten joined the committee late in life, and it is said he remained for far too long, being 83 years old when he retired and was one of a number who played no real role in the committee. Towards the end he turned up at meetings in dressing gown and slippers and smoked cigars.

Frauds, Quacks and Impostors

THE TERM 'quack' comes from Middle Dutch '*Quacken,*' meaning to brag or boast, promoting fraudulent or ignorant practices.

It can be loosely defined as the practice of palming off falsehoods as medical fact by a person who pretends, professionally or publicly to have skill, knowledge, qualifications or credentials they do not possess.

The motive is not always for the purpose of financial gain, by conning or cheating, but often to concoct or contort facts simply to suit one's own personal beliefs or pretensions — one's ego.

Quacks succeed by preying on the doubts and fears of vulnerable people, promising the kind of medical certainties that science often can not.

Tell-tale signs of quackery include dodgy references, cure-alls, asserting that science doesn't know everything, medical testimonials or anecdotes, and claiming centuries of evidence in support of something.

One of the reasons we have and will continue to have quacks is the continuing evolution in health care. In the past there have been many deficiencies and uncertainties in health care because of the lack of scientific evidence. This allowed quacks to flourish.

In the gold rush days medical care on the field was dicey. Anyone could call himself a surgeon and use a handy knife to do an experimental operation. For example, a gold miner was shot in the neck and the surgeon showed his skill by keeping up his patient's strength and making sure he had nourishment: he bandaged pieces of raw steak to his stomach. Somehow that did not prove to be effective, so he started at the other end and poured wine into the man's mouth. That was not much better because the wine ran out of the hole in his neck. He got no fee. The man died.

In the May 1893 issue of the *Australasian Medical Gazette* there appeared the following statement titled 'The Paradise of Quacks':

> *'We must not however overlook the fact that there are a very considerable number of unqualified persons many of whom have had no medical training whatsoever, who practise medicine for gain in these colonies. In New South Wales alone which has been styled the "Paradise of Quacks' we have upwards of 200 of such persons or one to three in proportion to registered men in active practice. Melbourne and suburbs can boast of 14 so called "Chinese Doctors" who reside within the boundaries of 'Greater Melbourne'. These irregular medical practitioners of all nationalities are found in every part of Australia though nowhere in such astonishing numbers as in New South Wales. The advertisements of these people are inserted daily in newspapers, the conductors of which assume themselves to be the leaders of public thought in the colony and are the means by which many suffering people are robbed of their hard-earned money in a vain pursuit of health from a source which is malevolently impotent for the purpose'.*

This is the situation applying only a few years before Ratten's time and when there were already three medical schools established in Australia

Dr George Faithful

He was born in Calcutta and commenced but did not complete medical studies in Edinburgh, Scotland. He came to Australia and in 1885 he was a chemist in Bourke, New South Wales. Because of his prior experience as a medical man and his earlier medical studies he became registered as a medical practitioner under clause 3 of Act 70, the Medical Practitioner Further Amendment Act of 1900 which said;

> *'It shall be lawful for the Medical Board or its doctors to place upon a separate register the name of any person who has passed through a course of study as a medical practitioner in New South Wales during the past five years before the passing of this Act'.*

Dr Faithful was now legally registered as a medical practitioner, untrained and without a medical qualification. I cannot quite see how he complied with the Act, but these were the times. There were no problems with the medical profession, the public or the Government. He was in an area of need.

Not much later Ratten was 'legally' registered as a medical practitioner, also untrained and without a medical qualification. There were problems with the medical profession but none with the public or the government.

John Palmer Litchfield

Born in 1808, the son of a poor London surgeon, he was apprenticed as a dresser at the Middlesex Hospital, but never completed training. Becoming a journalist, he decided to emigrate to Australia but before going made acquaintance of the Secretary to the Lieutenant Governor of South Australia. He signed on as ship's surgeon in 1839 and on arrival in South Australia advertised his credentials and was appointed Inspector of Hospitals for the colony of South Australia without salary. He started an asylum and repeatedly petitioned the Governor to build a hospital, presumably to have somewhere to treat his patients. But he must have overdone things because the Governor decided to investigate his background and found no records of his degree and qualifications. His Heidelberg University diploma had been bought and all his documents of memberships etc were false.

Litchfield was incarcerated in the debtors' prison, returned to England, presumably after someone paid his debts, and went back to journalism. In 1853 he decided to emigrate again to Montreal via Boston.

As before, he soon made acquaintances with influential people, including the Canadian Governor-General. In 1854 he was in Kingston, Ontario, the home of the Governor General where he was granted a licence to run a private asylum. The Queens Medical School was opened and Litchfield was appointed one of the teaching charter professors. He held two chairs, Midwifery and Forensic and State Medicine. He was regarded as an attractive lecturer and popular with students.

Embarrassment ensued when Litchfield admitted that he did not practise midwifery but only lectured on it and that he and three other staff members did not have medical degrees. On 13th January 1863 they were all examined, passed and were granted MDs from Queens Medical School. He maintained a dual appointment with his full-time appointment as medical superintendent at the asylum for the criminally insane and after ten years gave up his teaching position.

When he died aged 60 on 18th December 1868 tributes were generous and it was stated that 'naturally psychological medicine was his particular study'. I think Litchfield was himself a patient worthy of psychological study.

With his shrewd intelligence, glib tongue, charming demeanour and impressive forged credentials, Litchfield could ingratiate himself with anyone.

Milan Brych

A refuge from Czechoslovakia, he claimed he could not bring his medical qualification with him. In 1968 he was in New Zealand and the medical board granted him an interview. He obtained work in the Pathology Department of the Auckland Hospital and in the following year was granted provisional registration as an intern and subsequently full registration. He became a registrar in the radiotherapy unit again at Auckland Hospital and later set up a private practice. At no stage was he required to sit any examinations.

Brych came to the attention of medical authorities when he made claims of an 80 per cent cure rate for the malignancies he was treating. His claim was that merely from a blood sample he could prepare and inject chemoimmunotherapy specifically tailored to the patient's malignancy. He offered no physical examination, pathology, radiotherapy, surgical backup or follow-up. Challenged about his treatment, he claimed that the medical establishment was persecuting him. An inquiry found he had no secret cure and was using conventional chemotherapy. He was deregistered in New Zealand, which he appealed, but after information was obtained from Europe that he had not even been qualified to enter a medical school, a medical laboratory had sacked him for faking results and he had been in prison twice, he withdrew his appeal.

He then established a clinic in Rarotonga in the Cook Islands and he continued his work there. Patients went from Australia, New Zealand and even the United States to consult him there even being referred by doctors.

Brych came to Queensland in 1978 and, like Ratten, had the support of a State Premier, Queensland's Joh Bjelke-Petersen.

A meeting was convened in Brisbane including the Premier, the Minister for Health, Dr Lew Edwards, a medical colleague of mine who was later knighted and awarded Companion of the Order of Australia, representatives of the Australian Medical Association and cancer experts. Brych refused to give details of his treatment and it seemed unlikely that a clinic would be established.

The Premier still wanted Brych registered in Queensland, but Dr Edwards settled the matter by tabling damning evidence in Parliament. Brych left Australia, returning to the Cook Islands before moving again to the United States. He was charged there with fraud and practising medicine without a licence and was jailed for six years.

Was Brych like Ratten? He had charisma, gave patients hope and threatened legal action when challenged. He skilfully manipulated the media with newspapers reporting his apparent cures, but not following up or reporting their deaths. He capitalised on the failure of the New Zealand medical board to properly evaluate his qualifications and training. Professor John Scott, Head of Medicine at Auckland Hospital believes 'Brych got as far as he did because the medical, nursing and allied professions ...had not been handling patients uniformly with the understanding they required and deserved. I fear that we have not seen the last of the successful cancer quacks.'

Dr Jayant Patel

A qualified doctor from India who had trained as a surgeon and had a Master of Surgery (MS), he was an incompetent and a fraud, becoming known as Dr Death.

He was appointed Director of Surgery at the Bundaberg Base Hospital in Queensland in 2003 under area of need registration. He did not have a recognised specialist surgical qualification in Australia, and he had to work under supervision. Very soon after appointment concern was being expressed, particularly by the nursing staff, about his practice, but the Hospital ignored them and even gave good reports to the Medical Board of Queensland about his work.

Patel was accused of incompetent practice with a high incidence of complications and death. The hospital allowed him to perform major surgery it was not equipped and staffed for and that he was not equipped to perform. The hospital allowed him to do it because its funding was related to the surgery that was performed. It has been said to me that there were other practitioners in the area who had worse results. As in many such cases, personalities come into it and from all accounts Patel's blustering and arrogant approach was a really aggravating factor.

In 2005 questions were asked in the Queensland Parliament about Dr Patel's performance and calls were made for his suspension. On 2nd April 2005 Dr Patel departed for America on a business class airfare paid for by Queensland Health. On 22nd November 2006 he was charged with manslaughter over the deaths of patients; a warrant for his arrest was issued and on 21st July 2008 he was extradited from America.

There were three inquiries about Dr Patel in 2005. The first was the Morris inquiry — The Bundaberg Hospital Commission of Inquiry. Before the inquiry was completed it was shut down after the Supreme Court ruled that there had been apprehended bias.

Anther inquiry was established: the Queensland Public Hospitals Commission of Inquiry — the Davis Inquiry — which recommended that charges of manslaughter and other criminal offences be laid against Dr Patel. The Minister of Health at the time and senior Queensland Health bureaucrats were blamed 'for allowing the existence of an organisational culture of secrecy and ostracising whistleblowers that allowed Dr Patel's misdeeds to go unpunished for two years'.

Dr Patel was charged with three counts of manslaughter and one case of grievous bodily harm and pleaded not guilty. He was found guilty on all charges and sentenced to seven years' imprisonment. His appeal was dismissed. He then appealed to the High Court of Australia who unanimously allowed the appeal due to highly emotive and prejudicial evidence that was irrelevant to the case laid before the jury, quashed the conviction and ordered a retrial. At the retrial he was acquitted of one of the manslaughter charges and the others were dropped because of a plea bargain, with Patel admitting to fraud — he had neglected to give his American background.

In America Dr Patel first worked at the University of Rochester School of Medicine, where he received further surgical training. Quite soon he was in difficulty and in 1984 he was fined and put on clinical probation for three years over his failure to examine patients prior to surgery. In 1998 because of complications and deaths related to surgery, his practice was restricted by the hospital he was working in and he had to get second opinions prior to surgery. In 2000 his restrictions were made statewide because of continued deaths and in 2001 New York state health officials withdrew his licence.

'Holding out' — that is, passing oneself off as a doctor — is still a criminal offence and there are occasional prosecutions.

Claire Louise Bolitho — 2006

She was charged with unlawfully practising as a doctor and five counts of unlawful wounding. A Melbourne pensioner who flew to Perth for a shoulder operation at an exclusive private hospital said she felt stupid after discovering that her surgeon was an unemployed truck driver. She had believed that she was under the care of the Mount Hospitals head of orthopaedic surgery. Bolitho seemed to know all the medical terms and described in detail what the operation would involve, right down to how many stitches the patient would have. 'She was convincing up to the very last'.

Mark Collier — 2004

A telemarketer by occupation, he was a colourful impostor who had a major depressive disorder and drug and alcohol dependence. He impersonated a general practitioner and treated more than 100 patients He pleaded guilty to more than 60 charges including assault at an Altona medical clinic in Melbourne and was jailed for six months. He had immunised babies, gave out 38 prescriptions, changed dressings on wounds and counselled a grieving widow during his four days of work.

Interesting Cases

MOST medical practitioners with 50 years' experience have interesting stories to tell. In my case I have attended a murder scene and then anaesthetised one of the bystanders who had a gunshot wound to the arm. I have been on duty for the four major disasters in Hobart in my time: the February 1967 bushfires, the collapse of the Tasman Bridge when it was hit by the *Lake Illawarra*, the Mount St Canice boiler explosion and the Port Arthur massacre.

Ratten was no different.

As reported by writer Pauline Connolly, a Sapper McRae was shot in the shoulder by a Turkish sniper in the landing at Gallipoli on 26th April 1915. The bullet had travelled to his spine where it had caused damage to the spinal cord and partial paralysis. He was treated at a military hospital in England before returning to Australia, where his treatment continued at the Austin Hospital in Melbourne.

In October 1917 Ratten began what became a feature of his career — using newspapers to promote his work.

An article read:

'Dr Ratten surgeon superintendent at the Hobart, performed a remarkable operation today, and apparently with complete success. Sapper McRae, when at Gallipoli, was wounded by a Turkish bullet. He was sent to England and attended various base hospitals but without getting better, and was then returned to Australia, being treated at the hospitals on the mainland, then ultimately coming back to Tasmania without being cured. His complaint was a form of paralysis.

Having confidence in Dr Ratten he went into the Hobart Hospital and was placed under the newly erected X-ray apparatus. The bullet was located pressing on the spine and today an operation was performed resulting in the bullet being safely extracted, and the patient's condition is very satisfactory'.

The general public believed that McRae had been cured of his paralysis when in fact his condition had not improved, and the family was under the impression that the bullet had never actually been removed.

This is the typical approach of the fraud: tell the dramatic story but never provide a follow-up report on the progress of the patient — whether the patient died or the condition worsened, improved or not, or if the patient recovered.

Ratten was the surgeon involved when George Carpenter, a notorious criminal, killed three people at Levendale near Swansea in 1922 and was shot in the arm by the police. The arm was amputated by Ratten and after it healed Carpenter was tried, convicted and duly hanged. Professor Flynn, Errol Flynn's father, gave evidence at Carpenter's trial.

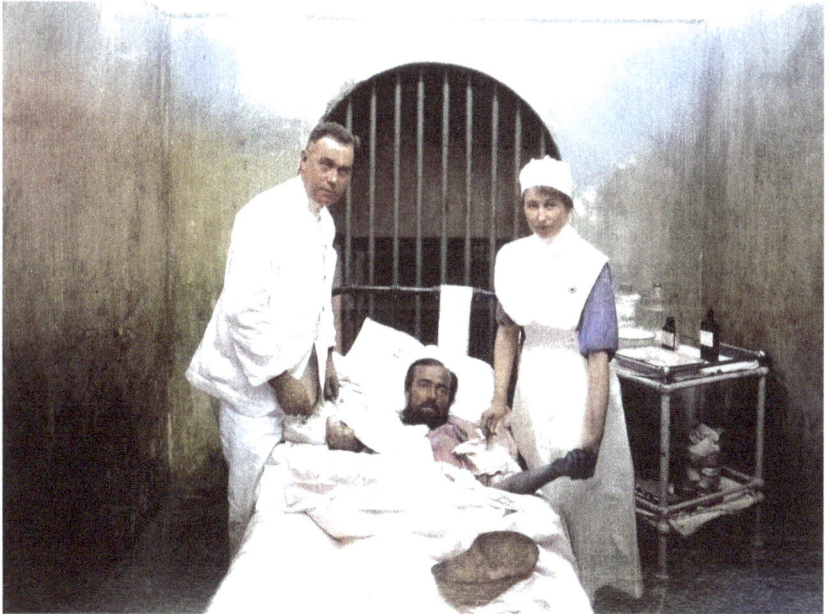

Ratten attending Carpenter in the Hobart Prison's hospital cell

Cyclist William Markham died when he was hit by a train and at the inquest Ratten said that death was due to cerebral irritation but two other doctors said it was caused by a fractured skull. These differing views led to the body being exhumed and it was found that there was no skull fracture. The coroner noted that the radiology expert had reported gallstones in another patient when they were not present.

In 1921 Chrisse Venn, a 13-year-old girl from North Motton, went missing while walking to the local shop; ; her body was later found concealed in a hollow tree stump. George King was charged with her murder, based mostly on circumstantial evidence, and was found not guilty. Dr Ferris, a contemporary of Ratten's when he was in Sheffield did the post-mortem and appeared for the prosecution. Albert Ogilvie was King's defence lawyer, and he was supported by evidence from Ratten and Dr MacGowan. Dr Ferris was found to have failed to carry out important forensic tests and this was deemed an important factor in the not guilty verdict.

Inquiries into the death ceased after the trial because the principal detective in the case, Harmon, was investigated and thrown out of the police force almost as soon as the trial ended. Harmon was accused of unfairly harassing witnesses and manufacturing evidence, though not specifically in the Chrissie Venn case. Much of the evidence against Harmon was compiled by Father O'Donnell (then in Latrobe) who had been involved in a dispute with the detective.

What is so fascinating is that all the individuals involved in this case were involved in some way with Ratten and the dispute.

It is not unusual for inmates of Hobart Goal to ingest foreign bodies of all shapes and sizes so that they can be admitted to hospital. Ratten had such a case which appeared in the newspaper under the headline 'Youth challenges digestion of an ostrich'. The inmate was operated on three times in five weeks. On the first occasion Ratten had to remove three three-inch nails and two needles; on the second, a fork and a five-inch handle from a tin pannikin; and on the third a large steel buckle, a piece of leather with three eyelets, a piece of wire nearly three inches long, a screw about an inch long with six buttons tied to a piece of string about seven inches long with another screw on the end.

Ratten appeared in several newspaper articles about bronchoscopies describing what he had done or commenting on what other people had done. A bronchoscope is a rigid tube which is illuminated and allowed inspection of the airways and into the lungs. It first appeared in 1897, so it was a relatively recent development and was gradually refined until 1966 with the arrival of the flexible bronchoscope, a major advance which allowed more detailed examination of the airways. When someone says they have used a bronchoscope to remove a foreign body from a patient's airway it can cover a multitude of situations, including such things as where and what the object is and how long it has been there. All these affect the complexity and seriousness of the procedure, which can be life-threatening.

In 1924 Ratten said he had, with the assistance of three other doctors, removed a pen holder from a patient's lungs using a bronchoscope. Whenever there was a report of a doctor in Australia or overseas using a bronchoscope, Ratten was quick to respond, saying he had done similar operations.

In 1946 there was a report of a child being sent from Melbourne to America with its mother to have a nail removed from its lungs. Ratten said he had done several such operations to remove peas and open and closed safety pins, but that he did not think that such operations had been performed at the hospital since he left.

In another report of the removal of a foreign body from the lungs, Ratten said it was considered miraculous in other countries but nothing out of the ordinary if it were done here.

In 1951 Ratten was still at it; when there was a report of a discharged .22 cartridge removed from a lung Ratten retorted that he had performed similar operations. Perhaps this was deprivation syndrome and a feeling of being a prophet without honour in their own country.

Could it happen again?

IT IS fascinating to contemplate whether such a situation could ever happen again in Tasmania. The answer is yes but unlikely — unlikely because an industrial conflict would not be allowed to go unresolved until the situation was out of control, the health of the community would not be put in such jeopardy because the registration process for doctors is now a vigorous one with many checks and balances and because of the increased sophistication of medicine.

Current requirements are that to practise a medical practitioner must be registered. This can be as a specialist which includes general practitioners, hospital doctors or in specified categories such as limited registration for area of need, teaching and research, and even as a medical student.

Once registered, the practitioner will have to obtain clinical privileges to work in any institution or area, and if it involves research, approvals by ethics committees and other authorities.

There are comprehensive identity checks, since in certain countries names can be very similar and confusing. There needs to be assurance that the person referred to in qualifications documentation is actually the person seeking registration, which can occasionally be a difficult and complex task. There are also 'present in person' requirements as part of the identity checks, as well as international and national criminal history checks.

All overseas trained doctors (OTD's) or those titled International Medical Graduates (IMG's) must apply to and have their primary medical qualifications assessed by the Australian Health Practitioners Agency (Ahpra).

Mandatory requirements include being able to communicate in English.

Assistance in checking qualifications at source can be obtained through the Educational Commission for Foreign Medical Graduates (ECFMG) — an American not-for-profit organisation that evaluates and certifies the qualifications of international medical graduates.

To be recognised as a specialist in Australia, all overseas trained specialists must in the first instance apply to Ahpra, which refers the applicant to the appropriate Australian or Australasian specialist college for assessment.

That body will advise if they recognise the qualifications and training of the applicant, if the applicant substantially complies with its requirements, or if it does not recognise the training and qualifications. It may grant fellowship and recognition or require the applicant to undergo further training or pass their examinations, or it may attach conditions to their practise as a requirement for recognition. Ahpra polices these requirements with constant assessment and review.

All other OTD's must pass the Australian Medical Council's MCQ examination, which can be completed overseas before arriving in Australia on what is called the 'standard pathway'.

They can then obtain limited registration subject to satisfying other criteria if they are working in general practice. There is a requirement to pass a pre-employment structured clinical interview (PESCI) for the position they propose to work in.

There are three pathways to full registration: pass the AMC clinical exam which has a very low pass rate; obtain a position — usually hospital-based — that allows a workplace-based assessment (WBA) which has a very high pass rate; or, finally, become a trainee of either the Royal Australian College of General Practitioners (RACGP) or the Australian College of Rural and Remote Medicine (ACRRM) and pass the fellowship exam.

Nevertheless, confidence tricksters still appear and have done until recent times; occasional examples appear in our newspapers. In consultative practice where medical procedures are not involved, it is relatively easy for the confident rogue to convince the naïve — and the not so naïve — that he or she is a medical practitioner. Just look at how many people are trapped by scammers today to appreciate the dangers.

All States and Territories have these problems. The greater problem today relates to performance and standards, particularly communication.

The registration of medical practitioners first became a legal requirement in Tasmania in 1837. The Colonial Parliament passed an Act to provide for the attendance of medical witnesses at inquests, a need at the time. As a result of that legislation it became necessary to declare who should, for the purposes of that Act, be deemed a legally qualified medical practitioner.

Parliament also resolved that it was expedient to regulate the profession and practice of medicine in Van Diemen's Land. Accordingly it passed 'An Act to regulate the Practice of Medicine in this Colony', 1 Vict., No. 17 establishing a Court of Examiners appointed by the Lieutenant-Governor, consisting of seven members including a president. Registration was granted following examination or letters testimonial. This Act took effect on 1st January 1838 and was possibly the first in the world to register medical practitioners and preceded the establishment of the General Medical Council, the equivalent body in the United Kingdom, by some 17 years.

Subsequent Acts were passed: in 1842 to amend and consolidate the laws now in place in this island regulating the practise of medicine; in 1908 the Medical Act 1908 which established the Medical Council of Tasmania; and again in 1959 and 1996.

In 2010 the Commonwealth Government, with bipartisan support, established the Australian Health Practitioners Registration Agency (Ahpra) which established uniformity of registration across all of Australia in all health professions. This had the added advantage of reducing the problem for professionals who worked in towns overlapping two States such as Albury-Wodonga, who had to register and pay both States' registration fees.

The Medical Council of Tasmania became the Tasmanian Board, Medical Board of Australia under the umbrella of Ahpra.

Fraud does still occur. Individuals can present false documents or genuine documents which have been granted not after a period of training and examination but simply for prior experience. Examples have occurred in my time.

One case was detected by the Registrar of the Medical Council of Tasmania while processing an application for registration. This applicant had previously been registered by the General Medical Council in the United Kingdom, their assessment being conducted purely on paper. The applicant had an American medical qualification and produced a registration document from the Texas Medical Board among other documents. The Registrar noticed that there were identical imperfections on the documents and suspected Photoshopping. In the applicant's presence she went to the Texas Medical Board's online register. There was a person on the register in Texas with the same first and last names, but the middle name and the date of birth were different. The registration number of these two people was the same. The applicant had stolen the identity of a genuine practitioner in Texas; when the registrar confronted the applicant with this, he promptly left the building.

The Department of Immigration, Multicultural and Indigenous Affairs (DIMIA) was notified and showed indifference. The applicant had been sponsored in Tasmania by an interstate recruitment company, as was common at the time, and they were horrified when they were made aware of the anomalies. When the applicant was later interviewed by DIMIA the sponsoring body was not required to be present. The result was that the applicant had 28 days to leave Australia unless he found a new sponsor.

The Texas Medical Board was informed of these events but did not respond, so the Registrar contacted the Texas Attorney-General's Department and the General Medical Council. The applicant was later registered as a medical practitioner in Botswana by the Botswana Health Professional Council but was suspended when the Council became aware of his fraudulent qualifications; he appealed to the High Court and won on a technicality.

The Minister of Labour and Home Affairs revoked the applicant's residence and work permits but the High Court again became involved and ordered a stay of execution pending a review by the court but prohibited his engaging in any employment. The Botswana Health Professional Council continued to investigate — sounds like the Ratten story— and, based on overwhelming evidence, revoked his registration. The applicant probably moved to fresh pastures.

In another case the doctor did practise in this State until the Medical Council of Tasmania was alerted by a medical practitioner about his competence. His registration had been granted under the Mutual Recognition Act, whereby if a medical practitioner is registered in a State or Territory of Australia, they can be registered with similar conditions in any other State or Territory. This person had obtained a medical qualification from a South American country based on prior experience — as a chiropractor. He had come to Australia as an overseas trained doctor, obtained the appropriate registration in New South Wales, passed the necessary Australian Medical Council examinations, transferred to Queensland under mutual recognition, joined the Royal Australian College of General Practitioners training program and then came to Tasmania. When the Medical Council investigated the practitioner, he immediately sought legal advice and left Australia at once. International medical organisations were notified. He is known to have established practice in another country and to have used the post-nominal FRACGP (Fellow of the Royal Australian College of General Practitioners) a qualification never conferred on him.

With OTDs there is always a conflict — on the one hand medical practitioners and medical organisations such as the Australian Medical Association and medical colleges insisting on standards for patient care and on the other the government and public demand for more medical practitioners in the community to provide an efficient service. Is it better to have an unqualified or bad doctor rather than no doctor?

Another issue is the use and abuse of the Medical Act — that is, interference or meddling by Government when it wants to achieve certain objectives or control, and which can complicate or inflame a situation. There are several examples which I can give over the past 50 years, some of which I can understand.

Following World War II there were displaced medical practitioners, mostly from European countries. Such persons were ineligible for registration in Australia and so Tasmania legislated for a special licence to practise here.

Licences were restricted in number and in the nature and place of practice and were granted following a period of supervised practice in a public hospital and passing an examination. The examiners were respected academics from established mainland medical schools.

Those who completed this supervised training and passed the examination were awarded the qualification of Tasmanian Licentiate in Medicine and Surgery (TLMS) and were required to work for the Tasmanian Government as a District Medical Officer for two years before being eligible for full registration.

In 1996, when the Medical Act 1959 was being amended, the Government succeeded in inserting a clause which validated the registration of several overseas trained medical practitioners who had practised in the State for more than seven years but who had failed to satisfy conditions that they pass examinations conducted by the Australian Medical Council. This move backfired. The intent was to keep these practitioners in the State by securing their registration and for them to continue providing medical service. Of the four practitioners who were favoured by this legislation, three immediately left the state and registered in other states under the Mutual Recognition Act, something they had not previously been able to do.

A further example of the Government seeking to secure the permanent registration of a practitioner who had failed to satisfy registration conditions is that of Dr Yastrebov, the Anglicised name under which he was registered. A Bill titled The Medical Registration (Dr Konstantin Iastrebov) Bill 1997 to grant him registration passed through the House of Assembly, but the Legislative Council deferred the Bill and established a Select Committee to consider the whole matter of the registration of overseas doctors.

The Committee reported:

'Having considered the evidence the Committee recommends that Parliament not be involved in the process of individual medical registration as it does not have the appropriate knowledge and experience.

If Parliament did proceed to deal with the legislation it would create a precedent allowing other doctors to avoid the proper procedure and to seek registration from the Parliament'.

The Bill proceeded no further.

The most recent intervention by government is the proposal to fast-track the registration of overseas-trained specialists.

At the time of writing there is a shortage of specialists in certain areas and the government is saying that the specialist college assessment process for overseas trained specialists is taking too long. They propose that the Medical Board of Australia provide a faster pathway for overseas specialists from the United Kingdom and Ireland, bypassing the College pathway. This raises the issue of discrimination against overseas-trained specialists from other countries. A similar decision some years ago was ruled illegal.

Since I started this chapter some months ago, this expedited pathway is now in place for general practitioners, anaesthetists and psychiatrists, with obstetricians and gynaecologists to be completed soon and general paediatrics and diagnostic radiology later in 2025.

The Last Years

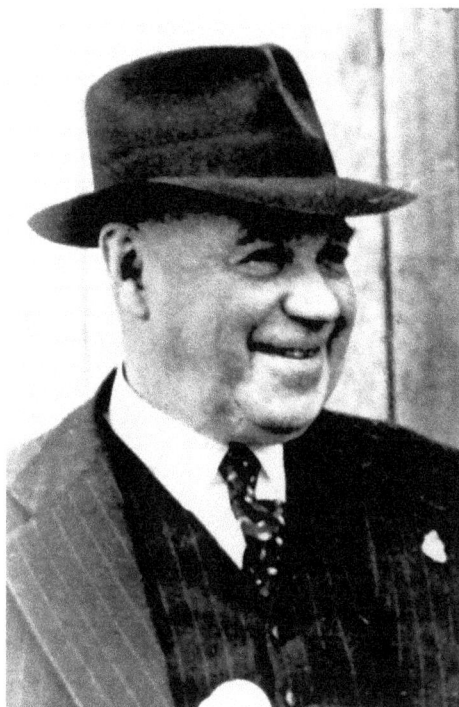

Victor Ratten in his later years

RATTEN remained a part-time surgeon at the hospital until after World War II. By this time he was 67 years old. During the war he was involved with army medical boards, was surgeon at the 111th Australian General Hospital, Hobart and performed camp duties until 1945.

This was quite a social time for him — it was his racing era. He regularly entertained on his launch *J'Attendrai* and attempted unsuccessfully to get elected to the Tasmanian Parliament.

J'Attendrai was a 62 ft (19 metre) luxury motor cruiser. It was a converted naval torpedo recovery craft (TRV *J'Attendrai)* It was bought in Sydney and the delivery was skippered by Don Muir. This was 1952 and Ratten would then have been aged 74. One of the crew was John Lucas, a marine surveyor who is now 95 years old. John, a life member of the

30 TON BOAT FOR LAKE EUCUMBENE

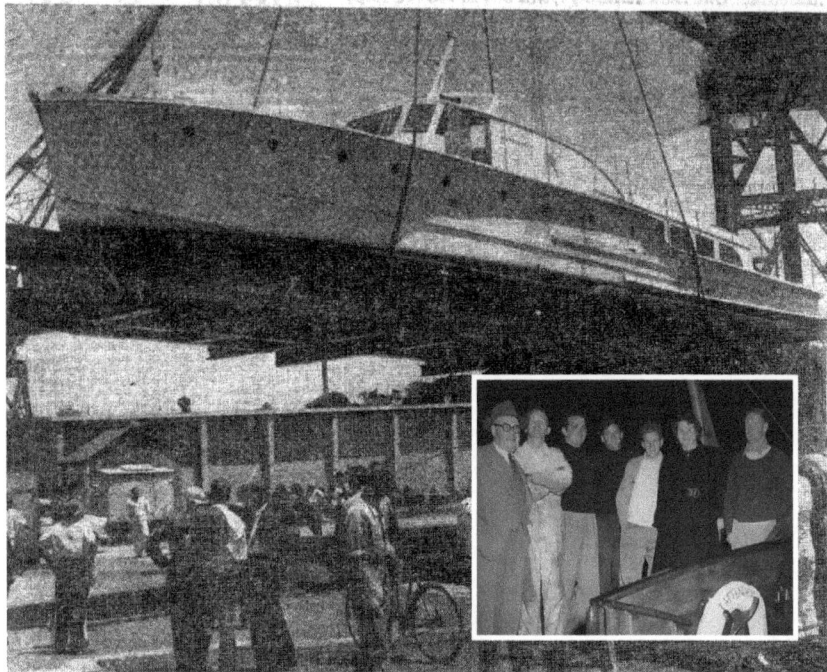

J'Attendrai is lowered on to a truck for transport to Lake Eucumbene, NSW, in 1959; (inset) A not very nautical-looking Ratten in three-piece suit and hat (left) poses with members of the delivery crew in 1952.

Royal Yacht Club of Tasmania, said that Ratten had no nautical skills or experience and the cruiser was always skippered by Don Muir in Hobart. Some of my friends recall their fathers being guests on *J'Attendrai*, the destination often being Opossum Bay.

The cruiser was later owned by ferry company Roche Bros or in joint ownership with Ratten. It was advertised as offering excursions to New Norfolk and was ultimately sold to the Snowy Mountains Authority in 1959 and used to transport passengers on Lake Eucumbene.

Ratten didn't change his spots in his latter years. He was in trouble with the Betting Board, and continued his publicity activities and a love relationship with the media.

Today, journalists would regard him as 'talent', knowing they would usually get something newsworthy from him.

One of his retreats was Huon Island in the D'Entrecasteaux Channel. Communication there was primitive — smoke signals were used to call a boat to cross to the island.

I assume that he gradually reduced his private practice and, as was the norm at the time, never formally or actually retiring.

In his latter years he was in an emeritus position at the Royal Hobart Hospital as a consulting surgeon and, defiant to the end, had his qualification listed in the annual report as MD (Chicago).

A significant problem was that St Helens Hospital was now in need of major renovations; the Government bailed him out by buying it.

He became increasingly frail and somewhat eccentric and was looked after by Dr Davis. He went to Tasmanian Racing Club committee meetings in his dressing gown and was reputed at another place to have used a fireplace as a urinal, explaining that he had an 'internal weakness'.

He remained a registered medical practitioner until his death on 30th December 1962.

Ratten died a reasonably wealthy man; his net estate was valued at £104,000, which in today's money is $3,585,000.

The Final Word

THAT IS the story of Victor Richard Ratten as I have ascertained it so far. He had some experience and training in health-related fields; he had a fraudulent medical qualification; he took advantage of an industrial dispute; and he went on to provide a medical service to the people of Hobart and Tasmania — but his presence probably retarded the advancement of medicine at the Hobart General Hospital, in Hobart and in Tasmania.

If both sides had been a little more reasonable — the BMA perhaps more so — there could have been a happier issue but the die was cast. One faction of the BMA thought the resignations were silly, wrong and ill-advised, and that the resignations were a blunder.

But the other faction was saying 'We will bring the government to its knees.' Premier Lee point-blank refused the BMA's demand. His view was that people had paid taxes for public hospitals and were perfectly entitled to admission and treatment.

Add to that a bitter press which boosted Ratten to an extraordinary degree and Ratten himself with his strategy of silence. The press played a great part in keeping up the antagonism of the government towards the BMA

The BMA was watchful and on the lookout for anything which could bring the situation to a head. This came when the question of Ratten's academic credentials began to be examined.

What remains fascinating is why the dispute and its resolution went on for so long. It was perhaps the result of a unique set of circumstances, like the Professor Orr saga or the current Save UTAS campaign; or maybe it was just Tasmania being Tasmania. Tasmania in its early days when it was Van Diemen's Land was different, one reason being that untried junior officers inexperienced in civil administration were sent to govern the colony. Good officers remained in Britain where they could get better positions.

This state has a reputation for getting national attention with issues that take years to resolve or are never resolved: issues such as the flooding of Lake Pedder, the damming of the Franklin River, salmon farming and the harvesting of native forests — or most recently, the proposed AFL stadium. Why do we have so many issues that remain unresolved for ages and bring so much attention to the state?

Is it our media? Is it different to that in other states? I don't think so. Is it because we have little else to talk about — or are we just seeking attention?

Are we naïve? Are we inexperienced in dealing with problems? Do we need outside help?

Are influential, noisy and controversial politicians part of the Tasmanian genome — politicians such as Michael Hodgman (the 'Mouth from the South'), Bob Brown the great green campaigner, the articulate Reggie Wright, Spot Turnbull, Brian Harradine, our only Prime Minister, Joe Lyons, or the new one on the block, Jaqui Lambie?

Is it the audience? Perhaps that is part of the problem. Tasmania has a small population — just over 500,000. We are over-governed with two Houses of Parliament — the Legislative Council, the upper house, with 15 members and the House of Assembly, the lower house, now with 35 members. As well, Tasmania has 29 municipal councils. Everybody has a say or expects to have a say and those elected to these bodies are desperate to get your vote.

Is it because of our small population people are more aware of issues and media coverage and opinion is more readily mobilised? We all know when something happens here and the public insists on its say.

Are we seen by other states as an arena for test cases, such as the BMA's use of Tasmania in the matter of wealthy patients in government hospitals?

But this is a whole discussion in itself.

It could have been so different. Ratten could have gone to America, obtained his MD from Harvey Medical College as he did, returned to Australia as he did, registered in South Australia and in Tasmania, established a medical practice in Sheffield, had his two-way ticket to Egypt with the Army, returned to Sheffield, relocated to Hobart and become a successful surgeon for the rest of his career with no one any the wiser. His mistake was to accept the surgeon superintendent position at the Hobart General Hospital when the BMA withdrew services.

All he would have had to do would have been to wait until the government had fixed the problem. But he accepted the position, the BMA investigated him, and the rest is history, as they say.

There were several other 'What if's'. What if the Royal Commission had ruled otherwise? What if people in the know had spoken up? Dental colleagues in Brisbane must have known that he had not undertaken medical studies in Australia and that he could not have done four years of full-time study or twelve years part-time in America to legitimately obtain a MD. He was away from the practice in Brisbane from September 1906 to May 1907. His father, the Reverend Ratten, must have known. If so, he was complicit.

Things quietened at the hospital when Ratten left but two issues remained — the honorary system and the consulting and private practice rights of salaried hospital staff.

The honorary system remained an issue, the belief being that the Board had little control over the medical staff. The government unilaterally abolished the honorary system in 1974 when honoraries were now paid for the time they were contracted to the hospital in what became known as the sessional payment scheme.

Rights of consulting and private practice for salaried staff have been a continuing issue until recent times. In the 1950s a pathologist, an anaesthetist and an orthopaedic surgeon were appointed full time to the Royal Hobart Hospital.

When they commenced, two of them found that there was a shortage of such specialists in Hobart, so they moonlighted and subsequently resigned their positions. The Hospital Board subsequently would not give full-time staff any rights of private practice, but this ruling was inconsistently applied, giving rise to much dissent.

To finish the story I must repeat such comments as these:

Amy McGrath/Cumpston:

'A very interesting story of a self-trained man who capitalised on Labor's natural dislike of doctors — an ingrained fact of Australian society since the earliest days'.

Robson:

'For his part the Governor Sir William Allardyce KCMG was quite satisfied that Ratten did not possess the necessary medical diploma required by the British Medical Association but also that if he had not shown great surgical skill the question of his qualifications would never have arisen'.

This is all I know at the moment, but it will not be the final word. More will inevitably come to light and more opinions will be expressed.

Ratten leaves a legacy of:

- A sign on his surgery door in Sheffield, *'Butcher Ratten'*.
- Gravestones with the words *'Killed by Dr Ratten'*, carved into posterity.
- A comment by Father O'Donnell, Chair of the Hobart General Hospital Board in 1936, describing Ratten as 'the cancer of the hospital'.

Ratten died on 30th December 1962 and his funeral was on 3rd January 1963. The death certificate was signed by Dr T Gaha and the causes of death were given as apoplexy, senility and heart failure. His granite gravestone is opposite the old crematorium at Cornelian Bay Cemetery.

At the service at the crematorium, Canon H C Cuthbertson paid tribute to the work of Ratten, who he said had served mankind with the talents which God had endowed him.

As with all this story, there are coincidences even at his final resting place. Less than three metres away is the gravestone of Dr Frank Fay MC, the BMA representative who negotiated the return of the BMA doctors to the Hobart General Hospital.

At its meeting on 9th January 1963 the hospital board noted with regret that Dr V R Ratten CBE had passed away since its last meeting. In the absence of the Chairman, the Secretary, Mr H Hope, had represented the board at the funeral and had forwarded a letter to Ratten's widow Blanche.

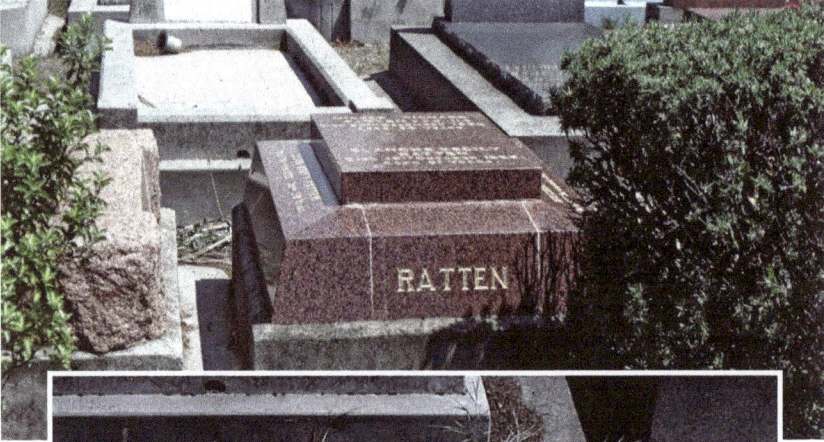

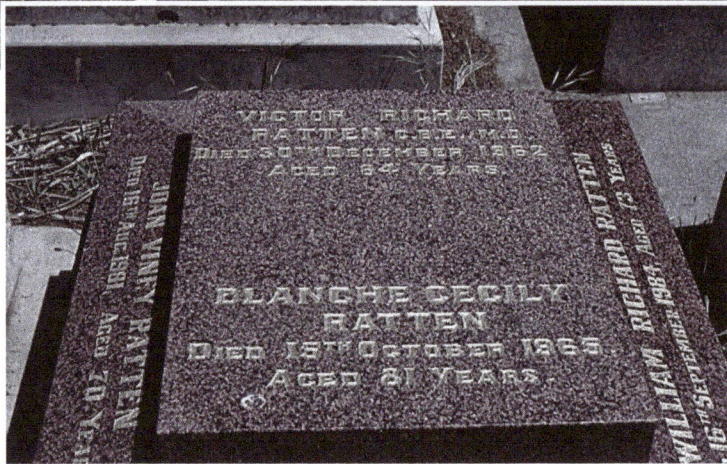

Appendix
The Evolution of Healthcare
and Healthcare Providers

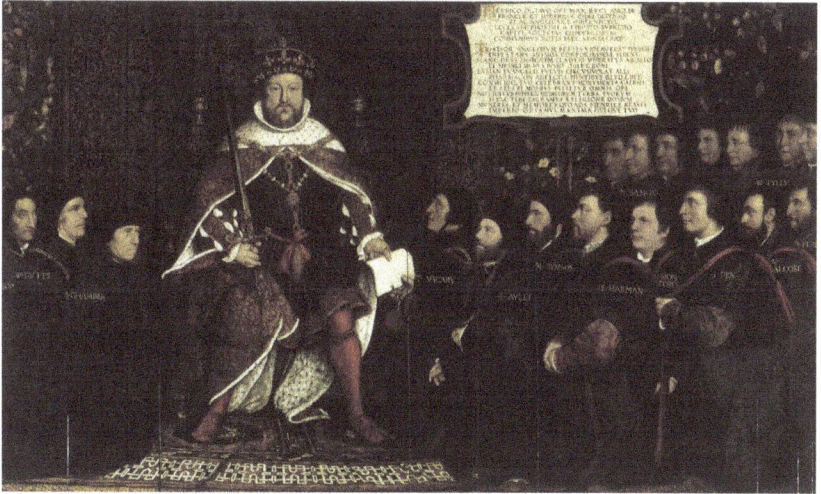

Henry VIII and the Barber Surgeons,
by Hans Holbein the Younger, Richard Greenbury and others

HENRY VIII is regarded by many as the originator of the regulation of medicine with his recognition of barber surgeons.

In telling the Ratten story it is important to relate his practice against accepted prevailing practice and standards at the time. Health care is continuously evolving, as is the question of who provides it.

In 1846 the first anaesthetic for a surgery was administered by Morton in Boston, Massachusetts on 16th October. The first anaesthetic given in Australia was by Russ William Pugh in Launceston on 7th June 1847. For the next 100 years anaesthetics were given by anybody with an interest or by necessity. This could include medical practitioners, nurses, lay personnel such as army medical corps — in effect, anybody.

Today it is expected that an anaesthetic is given by a medical practitioner, a medical practitioner with an interest or a contemporary specialist anaesthetist. When I had my tonsils out in 1950 the anaesthetic was probably given by a doctor in their first year out of medical school. In my final year as a medical student in 1964 I was required to give six supervised anaesthetics before graduating.

It was only in 1934 that interest in developing anaesthetics as a medical specialty in Australia started with the establishment of the Australian Society of Anaesthetists following a meeting at Hadley's Hotel in Hobart. The Society was established to look after the professional interests of practitioners giving anaesthetics, but it was not involved in training or examining. In 1952 the Faculty of Anaesthetists in the Royal Australasian College of Surgeons was formed, establishing the training and examining body in anaesthetics. To become a specialist anaesthetist today requires that you be a medical graduate, undertake two years of general training then five years of supervised training in approved and accredited positions, passing two examinations, one in the basic medical sciences and one in the practice of anaesthesia. Anaesthetists are required to keep up to date, undertake continuing education and to audit their work.

Orthodox practitioners follow evidence-based medicine but because there are still unknowns complementary or alternate medicine continue to exist.

Similar evolution has occurred in nearly all other health professions, all with the same structure involving training, examination, accreditation and continuing education. They are registered and legally protected.

The situation was very different 150 years ago, about the time Ratten was born. There was virtually no structured healthcare; values and beliefs were less scientific and a substantial part of healthcare was provided outside orthodox medicine in a diverse and flexible health care market. Medical history has been sadly misrepresented, oversimplified and many dubious practices have been seen as legitimate.

There is much more to the story. Between the extremes of today and yesteryear there has been a long process of change in who provides your healthcare for various reasons, such as where you live, access to orthodox practitioners and wealth. Other providers filled in the gaps.

A fraud is a fraud. A quack is a quack. They are not providers of the alternative health care which we have retained by necessity.

The real evolution to today's system began in the 1800s with the struggle for dominance by orthodox medicine. Its advocates believed they were right and promoted scientific evidence-based medicine where they could, aided by discoveries such as X-rays and the germ theory.

Orthodox medicine often lumped alternate practitioners together with quacks and frauds, which made it easier to argue their case.

Health care was in transition. Professional boundaries had not yet been drawn up and ethical guidelines were contested. Registered medical practitioners were at a competitive disadvantage because of professional restraints and sought protection through regulatory legislation. There was a correlation between the concentration of registered medical practitioners and action taken against alternate providers.

There is both art and a science in medicine and the provision of health care will continue to evolve. The range of health care providers in the 19th century was categorised by Martyr and in many ways still applies today:

■ Lay providers who self-prescribe, use patent medicines or homeopathy.
■ Lay practitioners who use a particular form of therapy to earn their living but who were not trained, qualified or registered such as masseurs and midwives.
■ Orthodox providers but who were non-medical such as dentists, chemists and druggists.
■ Orthodox unregistered providers such as doctors whose qualifications were not recognised or registered unorthodox medical practitioners such as trained homeopaths.
■ Orthodox and registered medical practitioners.

Even today distrust of orthodox medicine persists and many people support naturopathy, chiropractic and other alternate therapies. In the mid-19th Century the prevailing view was that you had to be a British medical graduate and perhaps that was because that was all we knew.

With the formalisation of medical education, training and examinations in most countries it has become easier to accept medical practitioners from other countries.

These days we admit there are deficiencies in our knowledge and we accept alternate or complementary medicine to fill the gaps in our care.

Today the spectrum of practitioners in medicine can include the formally qualified and trained, the formally trained and incompetent and the formally trained and fraudulent. And there are still the unqualified with little or no training — both are frauds.

This has created pressures to formalise medical education, insist on evidence-based medicine and better regulation of the medical profession.

This evolution was evident in Ratten's time in Sheffield. A gravestone in a Sheffield cemetery reads: 'William Henry Overton 1858-1920. Husband of Grace. Known as "Dr" Overton for his work in herbal medicine.' This cemetery, established in 1895, incorporated the earlier Sheffield Pioneer Cemetery.

The battle for dominance between healthcare providers continues and recently a book has been published in America — *Impostor Doctors. The Rise of the Nurse Practitioner and Physician Assistants in Health.*

A note on sources

THE SOURCES for this book have been gathered over some 40 years. Initially Professor Rimmer's book *A Portrait of a Hospital* supplied the background information about Ratten and the dispute. This was supplemented by reviewing the *Medical Journal of Australia* which extensively covered the saga. Many other sources were accessed as the story developed.

A Companion of the History of Medicine in Australia 1788-1939. A J Proust.

A History of Tasmania. Volume 11 *Colony and the State from 1856 to the 1980s.* Lloyd Robson.

A Port Fairy Childhood. 1849/60. Margaret Emily Brown.

Albert Ogilvie and Stymie Gaha — World Wise Tasmanians. Michael Roe.

American Medical Education. The Formative Years 1765-1910. Martin Kaufman.

Army records.

Australian Dictionary of Biography.

Australian Doctor 17 April 1998.

Dying to be Healthy. Alan F Dyer.

History of Medical Organisations in Australia. PhD thesis. Amy McGrath/Cumpston.

Impostor Doctors. The Rise of the Nurse Practitioner and Physician Assistants in Health Care. Dr Rebekah Bernard and Dr Nifan Al-Agba

Learning to heal. The Development of American Medical Education. Kenneth M Ludmerer.

Life over Death. Tasmania and Tuberculosis. Michael Roe.

Medical History Australia. August 2004.

Medical Journal of Australia.

Men of Influence. A History of the Tasmanian Racing Club.125 Years. 1874-1999.
Bertram Wicks.

Obliged to Submit. Wives and Mistresses of Colonial Governors.
Alison Alexander. Montpelier Press.

Official history of the Australian Army Medical Services 1914-18. Vol 1. A G Butler.
Pauline Connolly website.

Portrait of a Hospital. W G Rimmer.

Seeds of a Settlement. Buildings and Inhabitants of Belfast,
Port Fairy in the Nineteenth Century. Marten A Syme.

Sheffield Murals. Tasmania's outdoor Art Gallery.

'No Paradise for Quacks.' *Tasmanian Historical Studies. Vol 5.2 1997.*

Nineteenth Century Healthcare in Tasmania. P J Martyr.

The Pioneer Rattens of two Continents. Australia and North America.
Rosamond Barber.

The Sheffield School 1884-1984. B. Argent, D. Barker, H C Williams, D B Williams
eds.

The Companion to Tasmanian History. Alison Alexander ed.

The First AIF. A Study of its Recruitment 1914-1918. L L Robson.

The First 100 Years. Launceston General Hospital. Clifford Craig.

The British Medical Association and the Hospital Crisis. Rebekah McWhirter.
THRA Vol 52, no.3 September 2005

The Rivers Run Free. Geoff Law.

They Loved Him to Death. Australian Prime Minister Honest Joe Lyons.
Brendon Lyons.

Time to Heal. American Medical Education from the Turn of the Century to the Era of
Managed Care. Kenneth M Ludmerer.

'Victor Richard Ratten.' Michael Hodgson. *THRA* Vol 52 December 2005.

Why Politics Doctor Dr Frank Madill.